Dental Implant Restoration

Principles and Procedures

Stuart H. Jacobs

Brian C. O'Connell

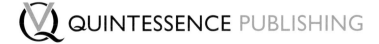

London, Berlin, Chicago, Tokyo, Barcelona, Beijing, Istanbul, Milan, Moscow, New Delhi, Paris, Prague, São Paulo, Seoul and Warsaw

British Library Cataloguing in Publication Data

Jacobs, Stuart H.
   Dental implant restoration: principles and procedures.
   1. Dental implants. 2. Dentistry, Operative.
   I. Title II. O'Connell, Brian C.
   617.6'93-dc22

   ISBN-13: 9781850971016

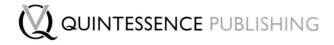

Quintessence Publishing Co. Ltd,
Grafton Road, New Malden, Surrey KT3 3AB,
Great Britain
www.quintpub.co.uk

Editing: Quintessence Publishing Co. Ltd, London
Layout and Production: Quintessenz Verlags-GmbH, Berlin, Germany
Printed and bound in Germany

Contents

Contents

Acknowledgements

The authors would like to thank Dee McLean for her invaluable assistance creating the wonderful line drawings, and Robyn Pierce and Lisa Adams for providing some of the component drawings.

There have been many dental colleagues who have provided us with invaluable advice and allowed us to show some of their cases. We are particularly indebted to Spencer Woolfe, Frank Houston, PJ Byrne, James Invest, Pranay Sharma, Ali Parvizi, Michael O'Sullivan, Johnny Fearon, Seamus Sharkey, Maire Brennan, Tom Canning, Maurice Fitzgerald, Padraig McAuliffe, Rebecca Carville, Nicky Mahon, Roberto Cochetto and Par-Olav Ostman.

We are grateful to Dr Richard Lazarra for agreeing to write a foreword for this book and to Biomet 3i for their assistance with technical information.

Finally this book is dedicated to our families, Jane, Adam, Emily, Anne, Ailis, Ellen, and Brendan, without whose incredible patience, understanding and tolerance we would not have been able to complete this project.

Stuart H. Jacobs
Brian C. O'Connell

Foreword

The purpose of this book is to give the dental practitioner, undergraduate and postgraduate student a basic understanding of implant dentistry and to provide an outline of the planning that is required to produce a successful aesthetic and functional result.

The scope of the text encompasses a general overview of the theory of osseointegration, the knowledge required to diagnose a patient for implant treatment and to plan a case. This includes the important interactions with surgical colleagues and laboratories. Much of the text consists of a practical guide for simple implant restorations using techniques that are currently available and commonly used.

The bibliography provided will allow the reader to further investigate the literature and to widen his knowledge. Implant dentistry is continually evolving and I feel that this book is a good starting point and serves as a foundation for all practitioners and students.

Sincerely,
Richard Lazzara

Introduction

This book provides the restorative clinician or student with a concise and easy-to-follow guide for the treatment of a patient requiring dental implants. It consists of two parts: Part 1 provides the clinician with a guide to patient diagnosis and treatment planning, and knowledge of implants and components; Part 2 describes practical protocols that will allow the clinician to carry out the restorative phase of implant treatment for tooth replacement.

Treatment of patients with dental implants requires the expertise of a dental team. This will include surgical expertise, which may involve a periodontist, oral surgeon or a trained general practitioner. The restorative component involves a restorative dentist and, importantly, a laboratory technician. It is essential that the team involved in the treatment of patients with dental implants works together to produce a treatment plan that will lead to an aesthetically pleasing and biologically acceptable final restoration. An example of an implant-borne prosthesis is shown in Figure 1-1.

Because the restorative clinician develops the blueprint for the definitive restorations, it is their responsibility to coordinate the treatment plan and lead the treatment team in achieving the best possible result. The position and arrangement of teeth will have a major impact on the number and position of implants that are finally placed. The optimum tooth position must be decided first and the placement of the necessary implants, or augmentation procedures, should follow. This "top-down" or "restorative-driven" approach is the most predictable way to achieve the result that satisfies both patient and clinician.

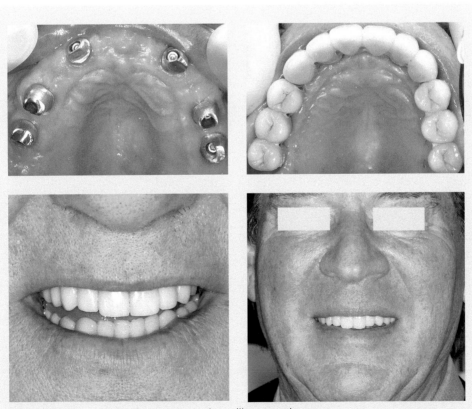

Fig 1-1 Patient with implant-supported maxillary prostheses.

In writing this text, the best available evidence in the dental literature was sourced. However, there is very little high-quality data, particularly in the form of randomized controlled trials, to support many common practices or products. In such instances we relied heavily on our personal experiences and those of colleagues to describe the assessment and treatment of patients. As such, we hope that readers will read the implant literature with an open mind and be prepared to evaluate and accept new practices. Many cases and techniques shown are based on one implant system. The principles are the same for most other commonly used systems.

Aims of dental implant therapy

The aims of dental implant placement are to:

■ place an implant into the jaw and avoid damage to the surrounding structures; these structures include the nerves, sinuses, teeth and periodontal ligaments adjacent to the edentulous space
■ achieve stable and bony integration of the dental implant
■ position the implant as close as possible to the long axis of the tooth it is replacing
■ reconstruct the soft tissue at the restoration site so that an aesthetic restoration may be constructed
■ maintain the interdental papilla to avoid unsightly spaces ("black triangle") between the teeth
■ facilitate a restoration that emerges correctly out of the soft tissue and is compatible with continued tissue health.

The aims of implant restoration are to:

■ create an aesthetic replacement tooth or teeth
■ maintain the soft tissues surrounding the implant to provide a natural and aesthetic setting for the replacement tooth or teeth
■ restore the form and function of the dental arches
■ maintain the occlusion
■ prevent drifting of adjacent teeth into edentulous space
■ provide a predictable and long-lasting restoration.

These are illustrated in Figure 1-2.

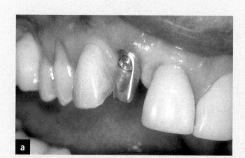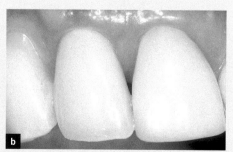

Fig 1-2 Replacement of a maxillary lateral incisor with an implant-borne crown.

Basic structure of an implant assembly

Two commonly used dental implants are shown in Figure 1-3.

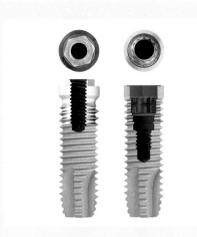

Fig 1-3 Most "root-form" dental implants have external threads that engage the surrounding bone. Internal threads are for the attachment of restorative components. Resistance to rotation is achieved by an external hexagon *(left)* or an internal hexagon *(right)*.

Threads are machined onto the implant, externally and internally. The implant is threaded into the bone (Fig 1-4) and covered with the mucosa (Fig 1-5). In the surgical protocol for submerged implants, this procedure is termed "first-stage surgery."

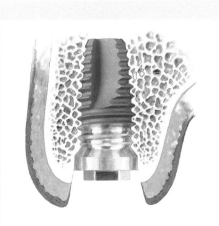

Fig 1-4 At first-stage surgery, the implant is threaded into the bony site.

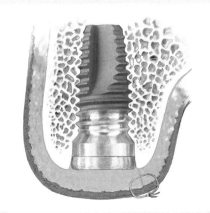

Fig 1-5 Once a cover screw is placed on the implant, the mucosa is replaced so that the head of the implant is covered completely.

After a period of non-loaded healing, the head of the submerged implant is exposed and a healing abutment is attached to the implant (Fig 1-6). This is termed "second-stage surgery". The smooth healing abutment supports the soft tissue during healing and facilitates restorative procedures by maintaining access to the head of the implant.

Once soft tissue maturation is complete, the patient returns to the restorative clinician; the healing abutment can be removed and the final abutment is chosen. The top of the implant is designed to accept the abutment, and the two parts are clamped together with a screw (Fig 1-7). The final restoration is then made and attached to the abutment by means of cement or a further screw.

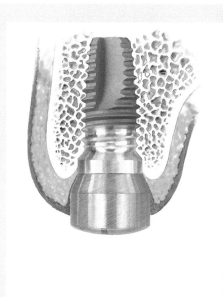 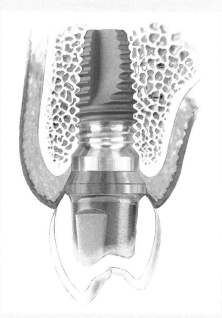

Fig 1-6 At second-stage surgery, the top of the implant is uncovered and a titanium healing abutment is screwed onto the implant.

Fig 1-7 Abutment and crown placed on the dental implant.

Some implants are designed so that the head of the implant is above the bone crest within the soft tissue. These are non-submerged or transmucosal implants (Fig 1-8). The principle of the non-submerged implant is to keep the implant–abutment interface away from the crest of the alveolar bone. Some studies have shown that this type of implant has improved soft tissue health and causes less initial bone loss at the implant–abutment interface than is seen with submerged implants.

There are many different implant designs available; the choice is based on the local environment, bone quality, bone quantity, and the preference of the implant team.

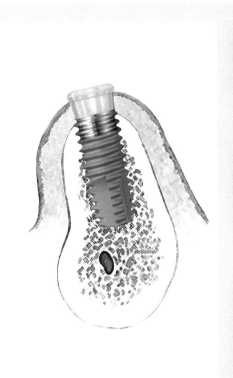

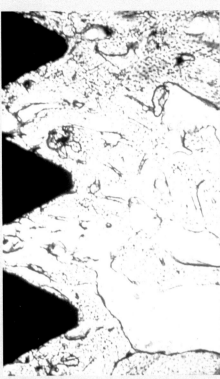

Fig 1-8 A non-submerged mandibular implant is placed so that the head of the implant is above the crestal bone. The implant may be just below, level with, or above the mucosa, depending on the thickness of the tissue and the aesthetic requirements.

Fig 1-9 Photomicrograph of an osseointegrated dental implant. Bone is intimately covering the implant surface.

Theory of osseointegration

Through an understanding of bone biology and wound healing, it was discovered that titanium implants could heal with a strong bony anchorage on which a fixed prosthesis could be supported. This concept of osseointegration was first developed in Sweden by Professor Per-Ingvar Brånemark in 1952. Osseointegration was defined as a direct structural and functional connection between ordered, living bone and the surface of a load-carrying implant (Fig 1-9). An osseointegrated implant should be constructed from a biologically inert material that has the ability to contact bone directly without any soft tissue interface.

Osseointegration represented a change in philosophy from other implant systems in which the bone–implant interface was variable and often consisted of fibrous encapsulation of the implant. Clinical use of osseointegrated implants started in the mid-1960s and, subsequently, has expanded greatly. In order to distinguish osseointegrated implants from non-integrated implants, the former were known initially as "fixtures." Research into osseointegration has continued and there is now well-documented evidence to support the concept. Osseointegrated implants dominate the dental market, and since the early 1980s several million such implants have been placed worldwide.

Factors influencing osseointegration of implants

General and local patient factors

While there may be few absolute contra-indications to implant therapy (Chapter 3), patients must be able to tolerate the surgical procedure(s) involved and have a good capacity for healing. Hence, implants may not be appropriate for patients with medical complications or chronic debilitating diseases. Specific factors to consider are:

- absence of infection — implants should be avoided where localized infection will prevent normal healing
- Radiation therapy — implants may be placed in patients following radiation therapy involving the jaws; this is a high-risk situation as patients remain susceptible to osteoradionecrosis
- good oral hygiene — patients should be able to maintain adequate plaque control around implants and the remaining teeth
- bone quality and quantity — there must be sufficient bone at the implant site to stabilize the implant at the time of surgery and during healing; integration of the implant is influenced by the quality of the surrounding bone.

Implant design

It essential that a dental implant is manufactured from a biocompatible material in order to achieve osseointegration. Most implants are made of commercially pure titanium, which is composed of >99% titanium, as well as iron, oxygen, nitrogen, carbon, and other trace elements. The exact composition of the metal varies somewhat according to the grades of titanium used by different manufacturers. A few implant manufacturers use a titanium alloy, which contains aluminum and vanadium. All titanium implants acquire a surface layer of oxide upon exposure to the atmosphere. This surface layer is mainly titanium dioxide and is normally less than 5 nanometers (nm) thick, although the thickness of oxide may be increased to several micrometers by processing the metal. It is, in fact, the surface oxide of the implant that the body senses and accepts as biocompatible.

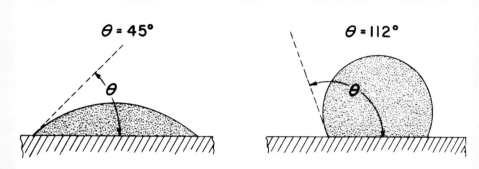

$\theta = 45°$ $\theta = 112°$

Fig 1-10 A wettable implant surface *(left)* has a low contact angle with liquids and promotes the spread and adhesion of biomolecules after placement. A polished implant surface has a higher contact angle *(right)* and is less wettable.

The surface roughness of an implant has a positive correlation with surface energy and wettability (Fig 1-10). Within an optimal range, a textured implant surface promotes the adhesion of biomolecules, stabilizes the blood clot during early healing, and encourages the attachment of bone-forming cells.

A roughened implant also has a larger surface area than a smooth one. This results in an implant that integrates more quickly than a smooth "machined" surface. The benefit of surface roughness appears to be particularly noticeable when the implant is placed in bone of poor quality. Manufacturers have used different processes to achieve a controlled surface roughness on their implants (Fig 1-11). These processes include grit blasting, acid etching, titanium plasma spraying, and hydroxyapatite coating. For example, acid etching an implant increases its surface area by 39%. Any implant treatment must result in a surface that will withstand functional loading without detaching, degrading or, causing an adverse tissue response.

Fig 1-11 Scanning electron micrographs of differently treated titanium implant surfaces (x2000 magnification): (a) machined surface, (b) grit-blasted surface, (c) plasma-sprayed surface, (d) acid-etched surface.

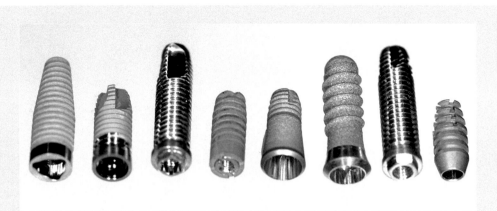

Fig 1-12 Endosseous implants have a variety of designs; they differ with regard to the taper of the implant, the shape of the threads, the extent and type of surface treatment, the type of anti-rotational feature, the height and flare of the implant neck, and the materials used.

Hydroxyapatite coatings are biocompatible and demonstrate good healing in poor-quality bone. However, there is some evidence that hydroxyapatite coatings detach from the implant surface, compromising their structural integrity. One potential disadvantage of roughened implant surfaces is that once they are exposed to the oral environment they accumulate plaque and are difficult to maintain. The rough surface containing plaque may promote inflammation and loss of bone around the implant. Implant manufacturers have developed a number of designs that vary the surface texture from one part of the implant to another (Fig 1-12).

Most commonly used implants are cylindrical or slightly tapered and have threads that give the implant initial stability. The coronal end of the implant is machined smooth to promote attachment of the soft tissues and inhibit plaque accumulation if exposed to the oral environment.

Non-submerged versus submerged implants

Two general philosophies of implant placement have developed in clinical practice. Either the implant is placed at or near the crest of the alveolar bone (submerged, Fig 1-13) or the implant is placed at or near the mucosal surface (non-submerged, Fig 1-14). Generally, the submerged implant is covered by the mucoperiosteal flap during the healing phase; after healing, the implant is exposed and an abutment is attached at the second-stage surgery. With the non-submerged implants, a healing cap, which emerges above the mucosal surface, is screwed onto the implant at the time of placement and so there is no second-stage surgery.

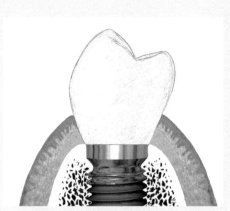

Fig 1-13 The head of a submerged implant is placed near the alveolar bone crest.

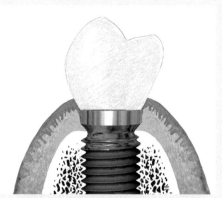

Fig 1-14 The head of a non-submerged implant is placed above the alveolar bone and near the mucosal surface.

Biologic width

Both submerged and non-submerged implants are capable of successful and predictable osseointegration. When the implant restoration is assembled, a microscopic gap exists between the top of the implant and the component that supports the restoration (abutment). This "microgap" is sufficient for bacteria to colonize and the resultant inflammatory response leads to crestal bone remodeling. Eventually, a "biological seal" develops around dental implants, which is a thin epithelial and connective tissue contact from the top of the implant to the level of first bone contact. The combined depth of the gingival sulcus, junctional epithelium and connective tissue attachment is known as the biologic width, as shown in Figure 1-15. The minimum biologic width around external hex dental implants is 3–4 mm. The establishment of the biologic width often leads to bone loss as far as the first thread of the implant; however, the eventual level of bone on the implant may also depend on the abutment connection design, location of the rough–smooth junction of the implant, shape of the implant head (cylindrical or flared), occlusal forces, and design of the prosthesis.

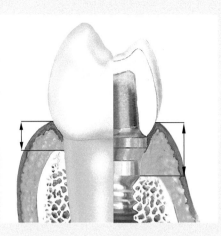

Fig 1-15 Comparison of biologic width around tooth and implant. The biologic width (shown by arrows) consists of the connective tissue and epithelial interface. This is generally greater around an external hex implant (3–4 mm) than around a healthy tooth.

The clinical implication of the biologic width is that there is typically more initial bone loss around submerged implants than around non-submerged implants. However, after the first year in function, it appears that bone levels are equally stable in both implant types.

There is usually a greater distance from the implant to the gingival margin with submerged implants than with non-submerged implants, so it is easier to create the desired emergence profile for the final restoration. Additionally, there is a greater risk in the aesthetic zone that a non-submerged implant will become visible if there is any supporting tissue loss after implant placement, as shown in Figure 1-16. This may result in the exposure of the top of the implant, which may create an aesthetic problem (Fig 1-17).

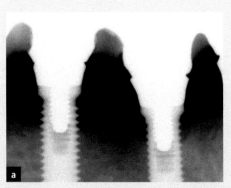
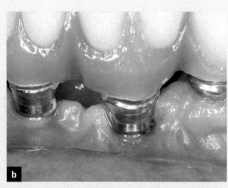

Fig 1-16 Implants where there has been loss of supporting tissue: (a) radiograph, (b) the exposure of the implant head in the mouth.

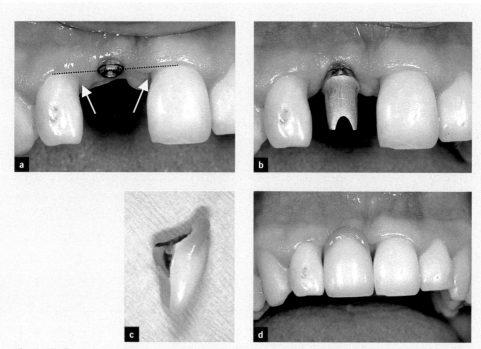

Fig 1-17 Exposure of the implant head creating an unaesthetic restoration. (a) Dotted line shows that the level of the implant placement is too superficial. Arrows show lack of interdental papilla. (b) The abutment screwed onto the implant, showing implant head and abutment collar exposed above the soft tissue. (c) The crown fabricated for this implant required a ridge lap to mask the exposed implant head and abutment collar. (d) The completed restoration showing the poor aesthetic outcome. The use of pink porcelain was not sufficient to compensate for the implant position and the lack of interdental papillae.

Platform switching

A recent modification of the implant assembly has been advocated to prevent the initial crestal bone loss that is seen at the implant–abutment interface when the implant is placed at or below the bone crest. By placing an abutment of smaller diameter onto the implant platform, the implant–abutment interface is moved inward from the implant shoulder (Fig 1-18). Hence, the microgap-induced inflammation, described above under "Biologic width," is further away from the crestal bone. An example of platform switching is shown radiographically in Figure 1-19. This so-called platform switching may better maintain bone and soft tissue levels around the implant. Platform switching may be particularly beneficial in the aesthetic zone where soft tissue preservation is critical.

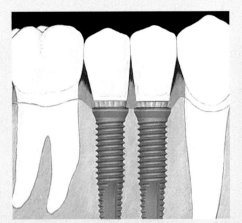

Fig 1-18 Platform switching, shown diagramatically, where the implants are restored with abutments of smaller diameter.

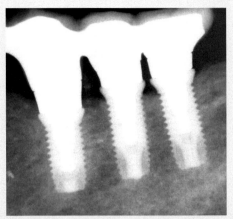

Fig 1-19 Radiograph of a restoration on standard abutments placed on wide-diameter implants. Note the maintenance of bone around the implant placed subcrestally *(left)*.

Surgical technique and postoperative care

In order to optimize the conditions for osseointegration, the correct surgical protocol must be followed. Excessive heat generation during the surgical procedure has to be avoided in order to maintain the vitality of bone-forming cells (osteoblasts) close to the implant site. Careful attention must be paid to flap design, wound care, and suturing.

The provision of good postoperative care by both the restorative and surgical operator will help to ensure the success of implant treatment. In the early stages this may include analgesia and antibiotic therapy, if required. The restorative clinician should ensure that there are adequate provisional restorations — preferably fixed restorations — that will not impinge on the healing soft tissues or compromise the stability of the implant.

It was originally thought that "early" loading of the implant — that is before optimum osseointegration occurs — destroyed primary fixation and caused implants to fail. However, more recent studies have indicated that it is possible to successfully load implants before complete integration. Nonetheless, it should be recognised that immediate or early loading is a departure from the standard technique and requires particular skill and experience, and careful patient selection.

Economics of implant dentistry

The cost of implant treatment is usually greater than that of conventional restorative dentistry. The increased costs reflect the purchase of components plus the need for surgical and postoperative care. Also, in some cases, transitional prostheses may be required and these have to be included in the treatment plan. Laboratory fees are generally higher for implant-related prostheses than for other restorations of similar complexity. The patient must be made fully aware of all these extra fees before treatment commences.

Many restorative clinicians, initially, find that implant dentistry may not be profitable, and this is usually because of a failure to anticipate all of the costs involved. In particular, clinicians often carry a larger inventory of implant components than they should. It is hoped that accurate planning, simplified treatments, and fewer components will make implant therapy satisfying and cost-effective.

Tips for cost-efficient implant dentistry

The following should be borne in mind to allow for effective pricing:

- check all costs involved before quoting a fee to the patient
- discuss all objectives openly with the implant surgeons and develop a good working relationship; implants placed in non-ideal positions cost more to restore
- use a minimum number of implant systems in the practice, preferably just one
- place a strict limit on the inventory of implant components and equipment
- initially, limit the type of procedure offered; start with one or two common treatments
- control laboratory costs; avoid handling fees by supplying components to the laboratory, or use preparable abutments
- include the cost of maintenance visits for patients following implant placement.

PART I

Diagnosis and Treatment Planning

Patient Education

Before embarking upon implant therapy, the patient must first fully understand the type of treatment they are going to undertake. At the initial consultation, it is essential that the dentist explains in detail the basic philosophy of osseointegration. It is very useful to have literature to hand to illustrate the types of treatment that are available, and this should be presented so that the patient may take it home and read it at their leisure. The patient and dentist should then have an opportunity for further discussion before making any definitive decisions.

Over a period of time, having treated a number of patients, the dentist should be able to build up a library of pictures that will clearly illustrate the results of implant treatment. The following are common questions that patients raise with regard to implant treatment:

What are the advantages and disadvantages of implant treatment compared to conventional treatment?

Advantages

Dental implants:
- facilitate the fixed replacement of teeth without involving or compromising any other teeth
- may replace teeth where the span is too large for a conventional fixed bridge
- can be used to restore free-end saddles with fixed prostheses
- are useful where there is inherent spacing of the anterior teeth (e.g. diastema), as the patient's natural appearance can be maintained with implant restorations
- may support fixed prostheses where removable dentures are unstable, unretentive, or cannot be tolerated by the patient
- can be used to improve the retention and stability of removable prostheses (overdentures) where fixed restorations are not possible
- have a good predictability and survival rate
- can maintain alveolar bone by functional loading
- may increase patient quality of life compared with conventional prostheses.

Disadvantages

Dental implants:
- are usually more costly than conventional prosthodontic treatment
- involve surgical procedures that may not be indicated for all patients
- may require extensive bone and/or connective tissue grafting
- require special surgical, prosthodontic, and laboratory skills
- require additional equipment and inventory of components
- may, with complex prostheses, be challenging for patients to maintain hygienically
- usually result in longer treatments than with conventional dentistry
- may give patients unrealistic expectations with regard to aesthetics
- may, if not placed precisely, lead to difficulty in providing adequate restorations
- abnormally shaped anterior prostheses may cause problems with speech.

How long does the treatment take?

The expected schedule of treatment should be discussed with the patient so that it may cause minimum disruption to their everyday life. Typical protocols are shown in Figure 2-1. In the mandible, the typical time for osseointegration to occur is 4 months. In the maxilla, 6 months or more may be required. When the implant is exposed at second-stage surgery, a further period is required to allow soft tissue healing to occur before restorative treatment can start. In aesthetic areas, 6–8 weeks should be allowed for the soft tissues to resolve. The prosthetic phase is then determined by the restorative dentist and this may take from 4 to 8 weeks, depending on the number and location of implants. Clearly, two implants in a single edentulous space will take less time to restore than several implants spread around a number of sites.

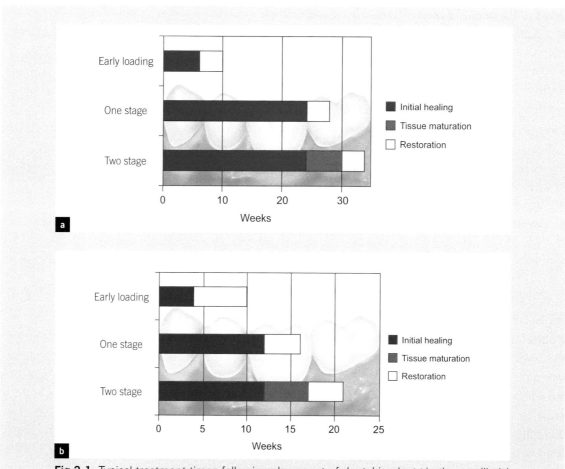

Fig 2-1 Typical treatment times following placement of dental implants in the maxilla (a) and mandible (b). Each case must be assessed individually and may vary considerably, depending on such factors as the initial stability of the implant and the need for adjunctive surgical procedures.

Recent research has shown that, in specific cases, implants can be loaded earlier than the classic protocols describe. However, more long-term clinical research is required in this area and the operator should first subscribe to the standard protocols before attempting early loading.

What type of surgery is involved?

An outline of the surgical phase should be given to the patient. This should include the length of time the surgical procedure(s) will take, together with an idea of how much surgical trauma they will experience. The speed of patient recovery will depend upon the number of implants to be placed, the implant sites, and adjunctive surgical procedures. However, there are very little published data to use as a guideline for patients. The patient must be aware of how long they will have to stay away from their employment. Finally, the dental team must discuss the options of local anesthesia, intravenous sedation, or general anesthesia. The type of sedation used may influence the amount of time the patient is incapacitated.

What is the success rate of dental implants?

Success or failure of dental implants has been described in many ways. While clinical survival of an implant may be construed as success, progressive bone loss around an implant may result in an aesthetic or functional failure. Osseointegration of implants may only be determined histologically, but this is obviously not practical on a routine basis. While various criteria for implant success have been advocated, in practice a simple set of standards should be achieved. In 1986, Albrektsson and coworkers proposed the following clinical criteria for implant success:

- an individual, unattached implant is immobile when tested clinically
- there is no evidence of peri-implant radiolucency
- there is less than 1.5 mm of marginal bone loss during the first year of implant function
- vertical bone loss is less than 0.2 mm per year, after the first year of implant loading
- there are no clinical symptoms such as pain or paresthesia
- there is an overall success rate of over 85% after five years, and over 80% after ten years for an implant system.

Implant designs have evolved since the mid-1980s, and as the experience of using implants has greatly increased, so have the expectations for success from dentists and patients. Certainly, there are several implant systems on the market that appear to meet Albrektsson's criteria for success. However, it is important to remember that osseointegrated dental implants were first used to provide fixed prostheses in the anterior edentulous mandible. Quite different success rates may apply to other sites in the jaw, such as the posterior maxilla, where bone quality is variable (see Table 2-1). Prosthetic treatment may also be associated with different success rates, for example fixed bridges, single tooth replacements, or overdentures. Hence, it is not appropriate to quote raw success rates for dental implants without taking into account the intended site and purpose of the implant. In addition, clinical implant studies are performed under a wide variety of conditions, with different patient inclusion criteria, various implant designs, and a range of follow-up times and success criteria, which are not always clear or consistent. Few of these studies provide high-

Table 2-1 Indicative dental implant success rates.

Implant site	Type of restoration	Implant success rate* (%)
maxilla	single tooth	97
mandible	single tooth	100
partially dentate maxilla	fixed prosthesis	95
partially dentate	mandible fixed prosthesis	94
edentulous maxilla	fixed prosthesis	89
edentulous mandible	fixed prosthesis	96
edentulous maxilla	removable overdenture	70
edentulous mandible	removable overdenture	94

*Median success rate of combined studies: Albrektsson et al (1986), Astrand et al (1999), Berglundh et al (2002), Brånemark et al (1995), Bryant et al (2007), Buser et al (1999), Ericsson et al (2000), Esposito et al (2007, 2009), Goodacre et al (2003), Gotfredsen et al (2001), Lazzara et al (1996), Moberg et al (2001), Pjetursson et al (2004), Torabinejad et al (2007) and Zarb et al (1990).

quality evidence to support implant use according to accepted criteria for randomized controlled trials. Dentists should carefully evaluate the data on any implant system they are intending to use.

When discussing with patients the overall successes and failures of implant therapy, it is important for the restorative dentist to understand the factors that influence the outcome of implant treatment. Clinical studies can only be used as a guide to predicting outcomes in an individual patient because it has often been observed that most failures occur in a small number of patients. As yet, we are unable to identify these individuals prior to treatment.

Many studies will calculate a prosthetic success rate for implant patients, which is usually higher than the implant success rate. There is little agreement on what is meant by prosthetic success, but often the continued use of any implant-borne prosthesis by the patient is deemed to be a success. This may not, for example, take into account the loss of one or more implants from a fixed prosthesis or the modification of the prosthesis. In addition, there has been less attention paid in clinical studies to ongoing problems with aesthetics, speech, or food stagnation. It often seems to be implied that implant failures "happen," whereas prosthetic failures are "caused" (by the dentist)!

Careful planning can reduce restorative complications, but will not eliminate problems completely. Patients should be fully informed of potential problems with implant restorations, and these should be discussed as part of the treatment planning process.

What is the cost of implant treatment?

The cost of implant dentistry is generally greater than that of conventional dentistry. This has to be fully discussed with the patient, and a written estimate submitted. Patients should be aware of charges for the surgical, post-surgical, and restorative phases of treatment. Many patients require a

Table 2-2 What fees for implant restorations should include.

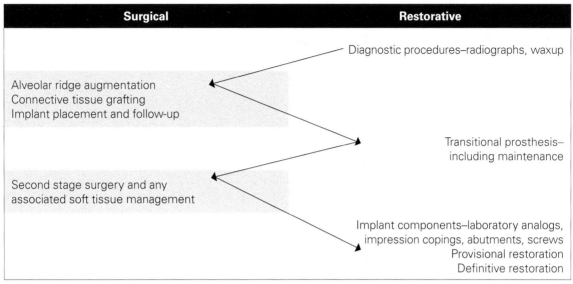

Surgical	Restorative
	Diagnostic procedures–radiographs, waxup
Alveolar ridge augmentation Connective tissue grafting Implant placement and follow-up	
	Transitional prosthesis– including maintenance
Second stage surgery and any associated soft tissue management	
	Implant components–laboratory analogs, impression copings, abutments, screws Provisional restoration Definitive restoration

transitional prosthesis during treatment and this should also be included in the overall costing. The definitive prosthesis will necessitate the purchase of components, such as abutments, screws, and impression copings. Laboratory procedures must also be included (see Table 2-2).

While implant treatment is initially more expensive than conventional dentistry, the predictability and inherent strength of implants may make these restorations comparable to other treatment methods in many situations. Nonetheless, maintenance or replacement of implants has to be taken into account when discussing the long-term costs with patients.

Not all cases will require all of the above steps, and the order of procedures may vary. This serves merely as a checklist to ensure that all possible costs are considered. The method of payment should also be clarified once the treatment plan has been accepted. Many patients prefer to stage payments over the entire period of the treatment and arrangements must be made before treatment is commenced.

Patient consent

From a medico-legal standpoint, it is mandatory that patients receive a written treatment plan, outlining the treatment recommended and the cost, together with a consent form, which must be signed by the patient and returned to the dentist before any treatment begins. The treatment plan should include all the possible risks during and after implant treatment. Patients must have the opportunity to raise any concerns or questions they may have before treatment begins, and should be aware of alternative treatment options. A template for the consent form is shown below (Fig 2-2).

I _____ consent to the treatment and costs outlined below.

Procedure(s): _____

(e.g. placement of two implants in the upper jaw; bone grafting; provision of implant-retained crowns)

Associated risk(s): _____

[Include general risks, such as pain, swelling, bleeding, and infection. Add the risks specific to the planned procedure, such as nerve damage leading to tingling or numbness, failure of the implant, damage to adjacent teeth, etc.]

Anesthetic planned: _____

[If using sedation, make sure the patient has been made fully aware of the risks and has been medically assessed.]

The proposed treatment has been explained to me by _____ (clinician), and I am aware of the likely outcome, costs, risks, and possible complications.

I acknowledge that no guarantees have been made to me concerning the surgery, results of the dental procedures, or a time in which it will be completed.
[Specify any particular issues here such as the need to undergo additional grafting, or the possibility of "black triangles."]

I have been made aware of alternative treatment options that are available and the reasons why this plan is the most appropriate one for me.
[e.g. adjacent teeth are not strong enough to support a conventional bridge; removable or partial dentures have been unsuccesful because of patient's gag reflex.]

I have been informed of the risks and likely outcome of not having the treatment carried out or completed.
[e.g. drifting of neighboring or opposing teeth, accelerated bone loss, etc.]

I understand that as treatment progresses, changes may be necessary to my treatment plan, and I will be consulted on these and my consent will be sought. I consent to my radiographs (x-rays) and photographs being used for the purposes of education, research, and publication.
[Specify your intention, e.g. to publish in a journal article.]

Signed by: _____ (patient)

Date: _____

Witnessed by: _____

[Make sure the consent is signed, dated, and witnessed.]

Fig 2-2 A template for a patient consent form.

CHAPTER

3

Diagnosis

A thorough analysis is essential for assessing the feasibility of implant therapy. Following the diagnosis, the dentist may present a treatment plan based on a comprehensive review of the patient.

Age of the patient

Age affects patient selection for implant treatment. Providing the patient is in good health, there is no upper age limit for implant placement. However, implants should not be placed in a young patient while facial growth is still occuring. Osseointegration implies ankylosis of the implant to bone, and hence the implant will remain in its original position as the patient's facial development proceeds. It is essential to wait until development is complete before any implants are placed. For most individuals this occurs in the late teens. Females generally cease growing before males. One exception to this may be in the anterior mandible, which is generally not a vertical growth center after childhood. Limited case reports suggest that implants placed in this area after adolescence maintain their relationship to the occlusal plane. However, it is usually advisable not to connect implants rigidly across the midline until growth is complete.

Medical history

Patients should be asked to fill out a thorough medical history questionnaire, to check their overall medical health. Patients planning to undergo implant therapy must be able to tolerate routine dentistry as well as the surgical phase. In addition to the standard medical questions, particular attention should be paid to the following points:

Is the patient under the care of a physician?
If the patient is under the care of a physician, the reason should be carefully investigated if there is a complex or unexplained medical history. Physicians, or other attendant caregivers, should be consulted about the patient's suitability for implant treatment. Patients should always be asked if they are taking any medication, as this is will often be a good indication of any underlying illness.

Does the patient have any allergies?
It is important to check whether the patient is allergic to any medication that might be used as part of implant therapy, such as antibiotics or analgesics. Metal allergies should be investigated to establish specific problems, by referral to a dermatologist for testing. Allergies to titanium are extremely rare, but some patients may have problems with gold alloys and other metals used in implant restorations. Patients with documented latex allergies should be treated according to the severity of their condition, using the appropriate non-latex materials.

Does the patient have a history of cardiovascular disease?

Patients should be asked specifically about a history of rheumatic fever or valvular defects, as antibiotic prophylaxis may be indicated for any implant procedure where a bacteremia may result. Prophylaxis regimes vary greatly from country to country, so practitioners must check the local regulations. It is best to consult with their general practitioner or cardiologist for advice on management of the patient.

Has the patient had a history of abnormal bleeding?

This should be investigated before surgical procedures are carried out. Patients on anticoagulant therapy may be able to undergo implant treatment, but may require adjustment to their medication, in consultation with their physician.

Are there any psychological disorders?

Psychiatric disease may contraindicate implant treatment if the patient is not able to provide informed consent or if the treatment would impact on their general mental health. However, many patients with diagnosed and well-controlled psychiatric conditions could be considered for implant treatment. The patient's physician should be informed of any planned implant treatment, and their advice sought.

Patients with psychological or personality problems can be difficult to manage clinically. Often these patients do not have a history of psychiatric care, but they may not cope well with implant treatment. Dentists should be extremely wary of a patient who expects their life to be changed dramatically by implant therapy. A history of frequent changes of physician/dentist, vague or atypical pains, or extreme anxiety about dental procedures or aesthetics should be a cause for concern.

It is often helpful to ask the patient to write down their problem and what they expect from implant treatment, in their own words. The dentist can then write down what can be reasonably accomplished by the course of treatment, as well as any possible difficulties or complications. Only when the patient and dentist are able to agree clearly on the aims and outcomes of treatment should you consider proceeding. Otherwise, the patient (and dentist) may well be disappointed.

Is the patient pregnant?

Pregnancy is not an absolute contraindication to implant therapy, though like any elective procedure, the placement of implants should not increase the physical or emotional stress on the patient. Diagnostic radiographs will be required and the patient may need antibiotic and analgesic therapy after the first stage of surgery. It would seem sensible to delay any implant treatment until after the pregnancy has run its full term.

Has the patient undergone radiation therapy?

Radiation therapy involving the head or neck will reduce the success rate of implant treatment, and the risk appears to be dose-related. Radiation reduces the vascularity of bone and its capacity to heal after injury. There is a lifelong risk of osteoradionecrosis after radiation therapy.

Is the patient undergoing steroid therapy?

Long-term steroid therapy may compromise the immune system and increase the risk of postoperative infections and delayed healing around the implant site. Any postoperative infection that develops during the early healing phase may have a profound effect on the ability of the implant to integrate. Poor bone quality has been associated with steroid therapy, which severely compromises the prognosis for implants.

Does the patient have diabetes mellitus?

Patients with poorly controlled diabetes have a higher incidence of implant failure than non-diabetics. The reason for this is unclear, but it may be due to delayed wound healing and susceptibility to post-operative infections. The controlled diabetic appears to have no greater risk of failure than a healthy patient. It is essential that all diabetic patients who are scheduled to undergo implant treatment have their disease monitored carefully by their physician.

Is the patient immunodeficient?

Patients suffering from any form of immune deficiency disorders should be treated with extreme caution. This group of patients will have an increased risk of secondary infections and a reduced ability to heal quickly after stage one of the surgical procedure. This includes patients with HIV infection, post-transplantation immune-suppression, or severe autoimmune diseases. However, if the patient's disease is stable, they may well be able to undergo minor surgery on the advice of their physician.

Does the patient smoke?

The significance of smoking for implant success is not clear. Heavy smoking may decrease the success rate of implant integration, according to early studies. The precise reason for this is not established, but it may be related to the fact that smokers may have a reduced blood supply to the bony site. Recent evidence suggests that if patients control their smoking during implant treatment, the success rate may be similar to non-smokers.

Does the patient have osteoporosis?

Osteoporotic patients must be screened very carefully before treatment is commenced. Osteoporosis results in a poorer quality of bone, leading to a compromise in the success rate of any treatment. Patients taking bisphosphonates will have poor bone healing, which may contraindicate implant placement (see below).

Bisphosphonate therapy

The use of bisphosphonates may contraindicate the placement of dental implants due to the possibility of osteochemonecrosis. This may lead to widespread necrosis of alveolar bone resulting in failure of implant integration and delayed healing and infection. Patients who have had intravenous bisphosphonates are at the greatest risk of complications, even some time after cessation of treatment. Great care should be taken in undertaking any dental surgery, including implant placement, in these patients and there should be careful consultation with the patient's medical practitioners.

Oral bisphosphonates, which are widely used for the treatment of osteoporosis, may not have the same implication for surgery as intravenous treatment. The risk to patients who are on oral medication may not contraindicate implant placement, but after consultation with medical advisers, great care should be taken if implants are placed.

Medical history: overview

None of the above medical conditions is an absolute contraindication to implant therapy. However, patients frequently have a combination of diseases, which may significantly reduce their ability to undergo implant therapy. Insufficient data exist to describe precisely the risk of each medical condition, so a degree of common sense is needed to determine whether the patient should have implants placed. This decision is also based on the extent of the procedure and the alternative treatments available to the patient. For example, a resin-bonded bridge may be a better option than an implant for a patient missing a single tooth and with a history of radiation therapy. On the other hand, it may be advisable to provide implants for an overdenture in an edentulous patient who has had unsuccessful conventional denture treatment, even if the patient has diabetes.

When communicating with physicians about patients, it is worth remembering that very few will be familiar with the details of implant treatment. It is helpful to describe:

■ the length of the procedure
■ the type of anaesthesia that will be used
■ any medications the patients will require
■ any likely complications.

For example, you may say that, "the placement of implants for Mrs. A will take approximately one hour under local anesthesia. She will be advised to take paracetamol as required, but no antibiotics. I expect there to be some localized swelling and mild discomfort, lasting approximately 72 hours."

Extraoral examination

As with all forms of clinical dentistry, a thorough clinical examination is essential to assess any patient fully. The main objective of the clinical examination is to collect the information required to arrive at a correct diagnosis and treatment plan. Detailed notes of the examination should be kept. Preoperative photographs of the patient are invaluable and should be a routine part of the patient record, as shown in Figure 3-1.

Any swellings or asymmetry of the head and neck should be noted. The joints should be checked for clicking, crepitation, and any other abnormalities. The orofacial muscles should be checked carefully for sensitivity to palpation. This may indicate a preexisting temporomandibular disorder, which should be addressed before proceeding.

All external areas around the mouth should always be examined for any abnormalities or pathological lesions.

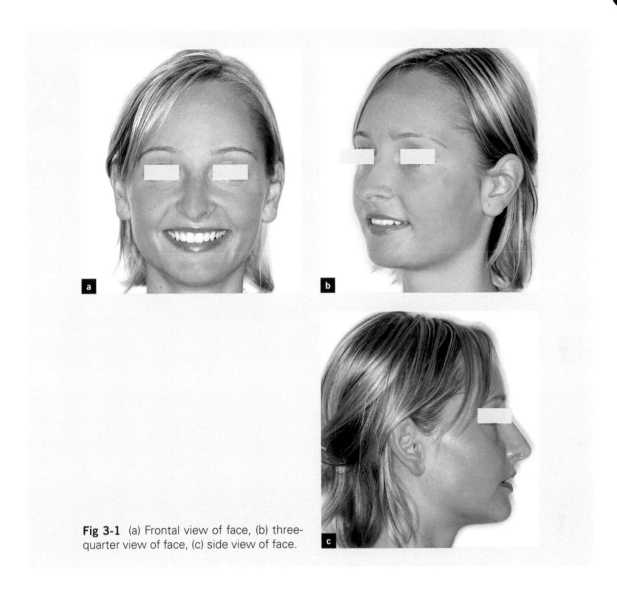

Fig 3-1 (a) Frontal view of face, (b) three-quarter view of face, (c) side view of face.

High, medium, and low smile lines

The skin and lips are first checked and the lip line recorded during relaxation, smiling, and laughing. The lip line can be classified in three ways:

■ high: the entire tooth and gingival margin is exposed during smiling (Fig 3-2a)
■ medium: the incisal one third or less is exposed during smiling (Fig 3-2b)
■ low: less than one third of the incisal edge is showing during smiling (Fig 3-2c).

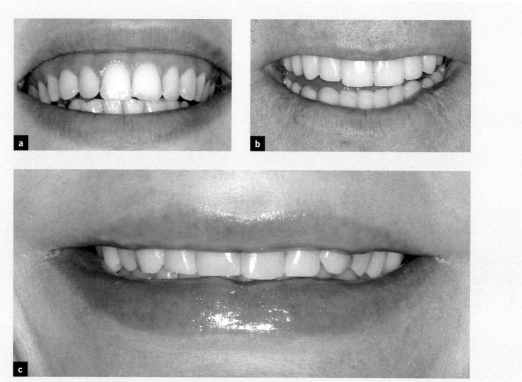

Fig 3-2 (a) High lip line, (b) medium lip line, (c) low lip line.

It is important to determine the normal view of a tooth for a patient, especially if the aesthetics of the tooth–tissue interface are likely to be compromised. From an aesthetic point of view, it is most difficult to achieve an excellent result in a patient with a high smile line. In this case, not just the tooth but also the whole soft tissue support is visible. Implant placement must be optimum and soft tissue management of the defect is critical. It is important that the restorative dentist and surgeon communicate clearly in all cases, but even more so in cases with high aesthetic demands.

Intraoral examination

A detailed intraoral examination should be made to identify any oral disease and to appreciate the local anatomy. The series of photographs should be completed to include the frontal view (Fig 3-3), buccal views (Fig 3-4), and occlusal views (Fig 3-5).

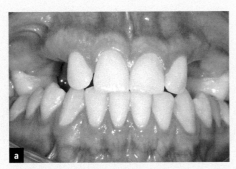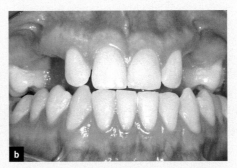

Fig 3-3 The frontal view of the teeth should show the anterior teeth in maximum inter-cuspation *(left)*. It is often useful to record a protrusive view of the anterior teeth *(right)*.

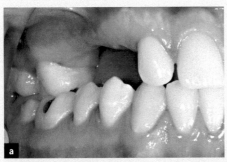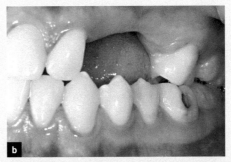

Fig 3-4 Right and left buccal views. The teeth should be shown in maximum intercuspation.

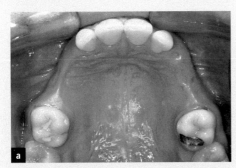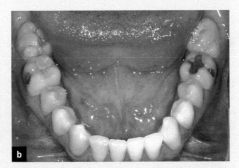

Fig 3-5 An occlusal view of each arch should be recorded. Standard views may be supplemented with local photographs of specific sites as needed.

Soft tissues

The mucosa should be examined together with the cheeks, floor of the mouth, hard and soft palate, and tongue for any signs of pathology.

Teeth

The purpose of the dental examination is to assess the health of the remaining teeth and which teeth should be replaced. Most practitioners would agree that implants should not be placed in the presence of active infection in the mouth. The status of the remaining teeth is important because, if their prognosis is poor, their loss should be anticipated in the treatment plan.

The teeth that are present should be charted, together with any restorations that are present. Any carious lesions should be noted, with a view to their treatment, before any implant therapy is started. Cracked or discolored teeth should be investigated. Endodontic problems should be treated as a priority. Any loss of tooth structure should be further explored in order to distinguish between attrition, abrasion, and erosion. Evidence of bruxism or clenching habits should be followed up.

Increased mobility of teeth should be documented. Mobility can be caused by periodontal disease, occlusal forces, trauma, periapical lesions, orthodontic forces, and naturally occurring short-root morphology. The causes of this mobility should be ascertained and treated, where possible.

Teeth that have tilted or migrated should be charted (Fig 3-6a). Not only may these teeth indicate the presence of periodontal disease, but they may also encroach on the space needed to replace missing teeth (Fig 3-6b).

It may be necessary to extract compromised teeth in order to improve the overall prognosis of the remaining dentition. For example, it may be better to remove periodontally involved teeth earlier in order to preserve and maximize the amount of bone that remains for implant placement. This may allow longer implants to be placed, and in a more ideal position, decreasing the need for alveolar ridge augmentation.

Occlusion

The occlusal examination is important in determining which teeth should or could be replaced by implant-supported restorations, and which type of restoration should be provided. The occlusal plane should be observed. Is it symmetrical on the right and left sides? Is the plane correctly oriented antero-

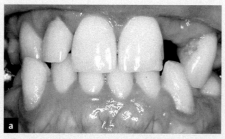
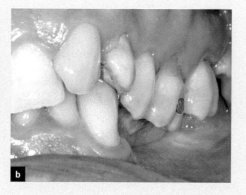

Fig 3-6 Tilted and migrated teeth should be noted, as they may encroach on the space for a replacement tooth.

posteriorly? Is the curve of Spee excessive or flattened? Are any teeth overerupted or infraoccluded? At this stage the dentist should begin to visualize how implant-supported teeth might be placed, and what effect they might have on the opposing arch.

The occlusion should be examined in the maximum intercuspal position (MIP). This position is the relationship of the teeth when the patient is asked to close together with their posterior teeth in greatest contact. Is the MIP stable? Does the patient move directly into MIP, or do they slide into the position? How many functioning teeth are present, and how are they distributed? Generally, patients should have at least 20 functioning units in their dentition. This allows the dentist to determine whether implant-supported restorations are required primarily for function or aesthetics.

The centric maxillomandibular relation (CMMR) is also checked. This is the position of the teeth when the lower jaw is guided, with the condyles in their most superior position in the fossae and with their anterior surfaces functioning against the posterior facing surface of the eminentia. Patients may be restored to the CMMR position when they do not have a stable MIP, for example when there are not sufficient functional units. Alternatively, if the occlusal vertical dimension of the patient is to be changed, the CMMR should be used for the restoration. Absence of a stable MIP often signifies the need for complex restorations that are outside the scope of this book.

The relationship between the upper and lower arches should also be noted, including any posterior crossbite. The anterior overjet and overbite should be measured, and the space for any missing teeth should be assessed at this stage (Fig 3-7). The presence of canine guidance or group function pattern of articulation should be documented. This demonstrates which teeth take most of the horizontal forces in lateral excursion and, hence, what type of force will be on the implant-supported restoration. Mandibular excursions should be checked for the presence of working or non-working side interferences.

Periodontium

The periodontal status of the patient should be assessed prior to implant therapy. Though there is no clear evidence linking periodontal disease to the failure of dental implants, it is generally believed that active infection should be eliminated. Studies suggest that osseointegrated implants may be

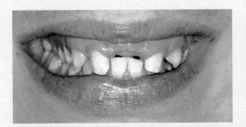 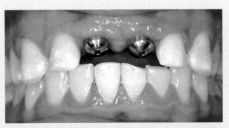

Fig 3-7 Static and dynamic occlusal relationships should be thoroughly assessed clinically and with study casts. Even before the diagnostic waxup, the space for replacement teeth can be evaluated. As in this patient, orthodontic treatment may be required before implants are placed.

colonized by the bacteria from around the natural teeth, and certain of these bacteria may accelerate disease around implants. It is advisable to treat periodontal disease, especially in close proximity to the implant site. It is worth emphasizing that the placement of dental implants will not reduce the susceptibility of the remaining teeth to periodontal disease.

Attachment loss (including furcation involvement) and pocket depths should be measured using a periodontal probe. Bleeding on probing and increased mobility should be charted. Reference should be made to the patient's previous records to assess the progression of disease. Plaque scores and oral hygiene procedures should be reviewed with the patient. Oral hygiene must be brought up to an acceptable level prior to implant treatment and should be maintained throughout the whole period of implant therapy.

Quality and quantity of bone

The quality and quantity of bone is very important for the success of any osseointegrated therapy. There must be enough bone at the site to place the implant in the optimal horizontal and vertical position as determined by the diagnostic waxup. In addition, the implant must achieve primary stability in the bone at the time of placement. Augmentation of the alveolar ridge may be required where there is inadequate bone to place the implant in the optimal position. Vertical augmentation of the ridge is more difficult to achieve than horizontal expansion.

When teeth are lost, resorption of the alveolar bone occurs. The rate and extent of resorption vary greatly. Five cross-sectional ridge shapes have been described by Lekholm and Zarb (1985), as shown in Fig 3-8.

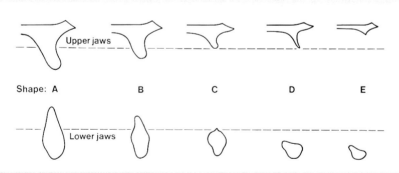

Fig 3-8 Classification of alveolar bone resorption and residual ridge shape, as proposed by Lekholm and Zarb (1985). A—most of the residual alveolar ridge is present; B—a moderate amount of alveolar ridge resorption has taken place; C—advanced ridge resorption has taken place; D—some resorption of basal bone has started; E—advanced resorption of the basal bone has occurred. (Permission for use of figure obtained from Quintessence Publishing Co Inc, Chicago)

Clinically, the form of the underlying alveolar ridge at an edentulous site may be determined by bone sounding. Under local anesthesia, a probe with millimeter calibrations is pressed perpendicularly through the mucosa until bone is reached to measure the thickness of the mucosa (Fig 3-9). Soundings are made every few millimeters along the lingual, crestal, and facial sides of the implant site, as required. The thickness of mucosa at each point is marked on a diagram or on a diagnostic cast. These measurements can be compared to the overall size of the residual ridge, so that the shape of the underlying bony ridge can be estimated. Bone sounding is quick, requires no special equipment, and is useful when a knife-edge alveolar ridge or localized defect is suspected.

Generally, implant placement will be facilitated where there is less resorption of the alveolus. It is useful to remember that resorption is primarily from the facial side of the alveolus, so this is the area that usually is deficient for implant placement. Resorption proceeds more rapidly in the mandible than in the maxilla, which means that it is often not possible to place implants in the positions occupied by mandibular teeth.

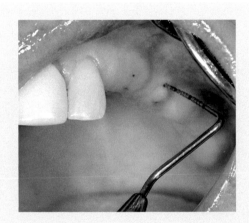

Fig 3-9 Bone sounding of an edentulous area.

Bone quality is impossible to assess clinically without drilling through the cortex to the trabecular bone, and so is often confirmed only at the time of implant surgery. Radiographs are also useful in the assessment of bone quality. According to Lekholm and Zarb (1985), the quality of bone can be categorized as follows (see Fig 3-10):

1. almost the entire jaw consists of dense homogeneous bone
2. a thick outer layer of compact bone surrounds a core of dense trabecular bone
3. a thin outer layer of cortical bone surrounds a core of dense trabecular bone
4. a thin outer layer of cortical bone surrounds a core of low-density trabecular bone.

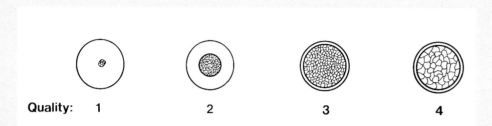

Quality: 1 2 3 4

Fig 3-10 Classification of jawbone quality (Lekholm and Zarb, 1985): 1. the jaw is mostly made up of homogeneous compact bone; 2. a thick layer of compact bone surrounds a core of dense trabecular bone; 3. a thin layer of cortical bone surrounds a core of dense trabecular bone; 4. a thin layer of cortical bone surrounds low-density trabecular bone. (Permission for use of figure obtained from Quintessence Publishing Co Inc, Chicago)

A great variety of both quality and quantity of bone is encountered in patients. Bone quality may vary between sites within the same patient. As a rule, type 2 or 3 bone, combined with good ridge morphology, provides the most favorable prognosis for implant therapy. The very dense type 1 bone is usually found in the anterior mandible and can be difficult to prepare for implant placement. Due to its lower cellularity, type 1 bone may have a reduced potential for osseointegration to occur. In type 4 bone, it is often difficult to achieve primary stability of the implant, which is essential for osseointegration. Clinical studies have shown that implants placed in type 4 bone have two to three times the failure rate of implants placed in the other bone types.

Radiography

Dental radiography is an essential part of diagnosis and treatment planning, in determining the overall health of the remaining dentition, assessment of edentulous spaces, and the final position of dental implants. Radiographs that may be required include: periapical, panoramic, cephalometric, and cross-sectional (tomographic).

It is important to remember that ionizing radiation is a potential risk—though very small—to health. This risk must be balanced against the diagnostic information that is gained from the radiograph. Diagnostic images are associated with a wide range of radiation exposures, as indicated in Table 3-1.

Table 3-1 Relative dose of radiation from various radiographic techniques.

Type of image	Relative effective dose*
periapical radiograph	1–3 per exposure
panoramic radiograph	1.5–10
lateral cephalogram	5
conventional tomograph	1–15 per cut (depending on the site)
computed tomograph	75–300 per jaw
cone beam image	15–25

*relative dose of 1 is 0.002 mSv. Large variations in exposure are reported for most techniques, depending on the site of the exposure, the type of equipment used, and the level of resolution. Adapted from Harris et al (2002) and Dreiseidler et al (2009).

Periapical radiography

Periapical radiographs are used to evaluate the teeth for any signs of disease and for surrounding bone levels (Fig 3-11). The implant site itself can be assessed for bone height, the mesiodistal space available, and general bone density and quality. It is also possible to determine the angulation and morphology of the roots adjacent to the edentulous space.

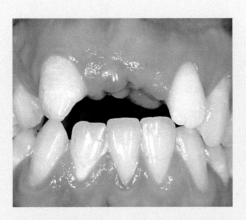 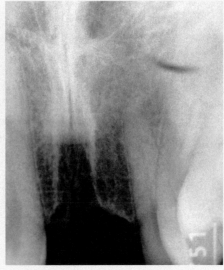

Fig 3-11 Clinical presentation and periapical radiograph of an edentulous space. The radiograph reveals a bony defect that is not apparent clinically.

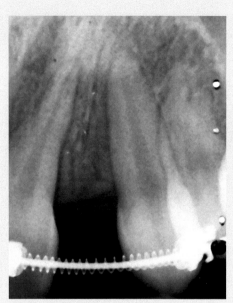

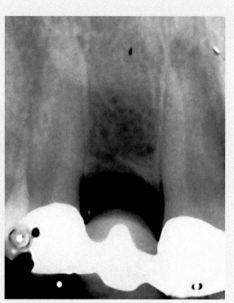

Fig 3-12 Periapical radiograph of an edentulous space. There is insufficient space between the converging roots for placement of a dental implant.

Fig 3-13 Orthodontic uprighting of the teeth was required before implant surgery. The space was maintained with a provisional adhesive bridge.

Convergent roots adjacent to the potential implant site might create a problem, as the mesiodistal space might look adequate, supragingivally, but might diminish apically (Fig 3-12). This will reduce the length of implant that can be placed in the site and may require orthodontic correction or the use of an alternative restoration (Fig 3-13).

Panoramic radiography

A panoramic radiograph may provide a very useful image for diagnosis in osseointegration therapy. This type of radiograph may show the presence of unerupted teeth, residual roots, or bony lesions at the implant site, and allows specific landmarks to be identified (Fig 3-14). This is especially useful in the initial assessment of the sinuses in the posterior maxilla. In the mandible, the inferior dental canals, mental foramina, and inferior border may be identified.

A major disadvantage of the panoramic radiograph is its level of distortion. Dental panoramic radiographs give a distortion of 50–70% in the horizontal plane and 10–32% in the vertical axis. Because of the distortion, it is difficult to measure implant sites accurately.

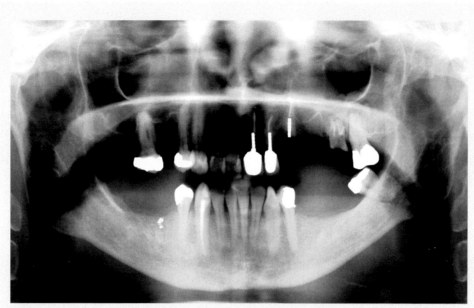

Fig 3-14 In implant diagnosis, a panoramic radiograph is useful as a survey of the remaining dentition, for the detection of pathosis at potential implant sites, and to estimate the alveolar bone in relation to the maxillary sinuses.

A diagnostic radiographic guide can be constructed with metal balls embedded at the site of the missing tooth or teeth. This guide is placed in the mouth when the panoramic radiograph is taken (Fig 3-15). The size of the ball on the radiograph is measured and compared to the known dimensions of the ball. The distortion factor at that location can be calculated using the ratio of the real-to-radiographic size of the ball. Using the distortion factor, the actual height of bone at the implant site can be calculated.

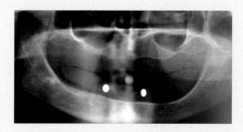

Fig 3-15 Panoramic radiograph with ball bearings used to correct for the distortion factor.

Lateral cephalography

A lateral view of the skull is particularly useful for the assessment of implants in the anterior mandible and maxilla. In this area, the alveolar ridge is often thin, and the body of the mandible has a variable angle to the occlusal plane (Fig 3-16). A lateral cephalogram will show if it is possible to place implants perpendicular to the occlusal plane or if they will be excessively inclined.

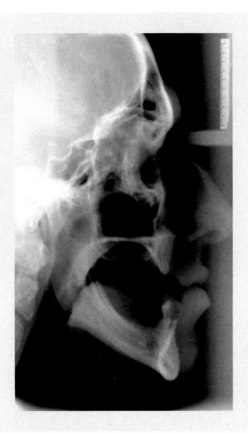

Fig 3-16 The lateral skull radiograph is useful for imaging the residual alveolar ridge in the anterior maxilla and mandible. In particular, the orientation of the alveolus to the occlusal plane can be visualized, which largely determines the axial inclination of the implants.

Cross-sectional imaging

Tomographs provide cross-sectional views of the jaws and allow for accurate assessment of bone volumes for implant placement. Tomographic images are very useful in showing a cross-section of small edentulous spaces (Fig 3-17). Such images may be indicated where there is a risk of damage to anatomic structures by implant placement or where there is limited bone available for successful implant surgery. A few selected planes, at 3–4 mm intervals, are usually sufficient to plan the implant placement.

Computerized tomography

Multiplanar reformatted computerized tomography (CT) can construct an entire three-dimensional image of the jaws, which may be viewed from any direction. The positions of vital structures can be identified and the amount of alveolar bone measured. From these measurements, the width and length of the proposed implants can be planned.

The ideal position of the implants can be related to the CT image by having the patient wear a radiographic guide during the scan. If radio-opaque teeth are placed on the guide in the position of the definitive restorations (based on the diagnostic waxup), the teeth will be visible on the CT image (Fig 3-18). The alveolar ridge size, morphology, and position relative to the final tooth position may be seen. It is then possible to determine whether implants can be placed in these locations or if secondary sites may need to be used. This process is also useful to assess whether augmentation of the alveolar ridge will be required.

When used with a radio-opaque guide, the desired tooth position can be seen in relation to the alveolar bone (Fig 3-19). This allows for implant placement to be coordinated with the prosthetic treatment.

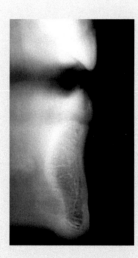

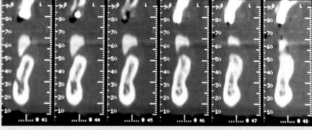

Fig 3-17 Selected tomographic image of an edentulous space showing a cross-section of the site for implant placement.

Fig 3-18 Computed tomography (CT) image showing cross-section of radio-opaque tooth placed over the mandible.

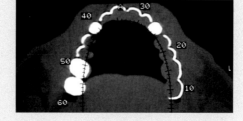

Fig 3-19 Horizontal CT image of radiographic guide placed in the maxilla.

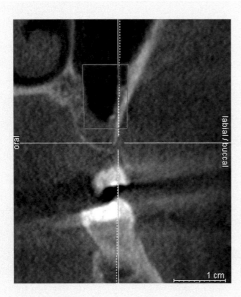

Fig 3-20 Section from CT scan showing insufficient bone present for implant placement in the maxilla due to enlargement of the sinus.

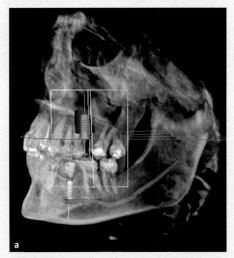

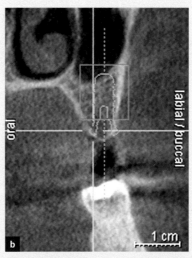

Fig 3-21 Three-dimensional image of the jaws based on a CT scan (a) showing the image of a proposed implant on the left side of the maxilla (b). In this way, the length and width of an implant may be assessed at the planning stage. (Courtesy of Dr. Anne O'Donoghue)

CT scans are most useful where several implants are planned near vital structures, such as the maxillary sinus, incisive canal, mental foramen, or inferior alveolar canal (Fig 3-20). The radiologist may be asked to mark these structures on the images (Fig 3-21a). Accurate images are also very helpful in the case of thin or undercut alveolar ridges, where it is difficult to assess implant sites clinically. It is

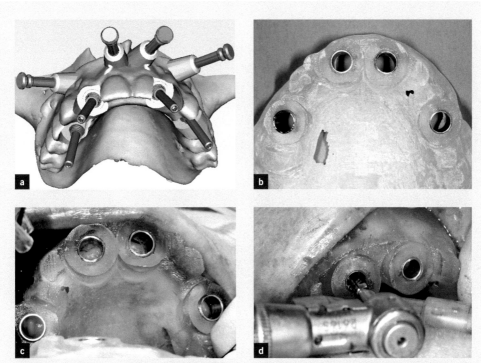

Fig 3-22 (a) Computer-designed surgical guide in place, which shows the orientation of the implants to the final restoration. (b) Surgical guide made with tubes to facilitate drilling and implant placement. (c) Surgical guide in place. (d) Drilling procedure using tubes in the surgical guide.

important that CT scans are oriented parallel to an appropriate reference plane, which is usually the occlusal plane. The dentist may need to provide guidance for the radiographer in orienting the patient.

Computer software is available that allows for implants of different sizes to be viewed in any position on the CT image (Fig 3-21b). This may help to visualize limitations of bone at a given site or the resulting angulation of the implant. However, it is not always easy for surgeons to place the implants in the precise three-dimensional position planned on the CT scan. Recent advances in radiological analysis allow for construction of a three-dimensional model that is a replica of the jaws. From this replica, a surgical guide can be designed that fits precisely the tissues or remaining teeth (Fig 3-22a). The precision of this technique allows the surgical guide to be constructed with tubes to direct the implant drills (Fig 3-22b). Hence the position of the implant is completely predetermined by the tubes in the guide (Fig 3-22c). Implants are then placed by puncturing the gingival tissue and drilling the implant sites without the need to raise surgical flaps (Fig 3-22d). This technique is less invasive and may lead to less pain and quicker healing times. The technique assumes exact positioning and complete stability of the surgical guide over the implant site.

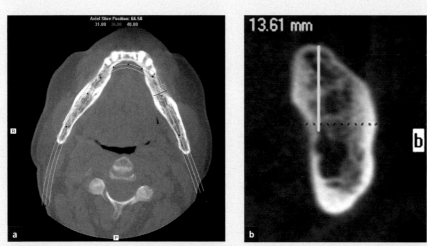

Fig 3-23 Cone beam computed tomography images. Software allows for edentulous areas to be visualized from any angle and for measurement between anatomic landmarks (b)

Cone beam imaging

Cone beam imaging is a further advancement of computed tomography, using a cone-shaped x-ray with an image intensifier or image detector. Three-dimensional images may be generated with substantially reduced radiation dosage to the patient. There is a significant cost reduction, which may allow the clinician to use this imaging within a practice setting. The images generated by the cone beam provide the same accuracy as conventional computed tomography for the location of anatomical structures and the measurements required for implant placement (Fig 3-23).

The radiographs needed to diagnose and treat an individual patient will depend largely on the scope of the proposed restoration and its anatomic location (Table 3-2). The restorative dentist should be able to collect sufficient clinical and radiographic information to devise a treatment plan for the

Table 3-2 Guide to radiographs for implant diagnosis and treatment.

Planned restoration	Screening and treatment planning (usually restorative dentist)	Detailed planning or presurgical stage
single tooth	periapical	periapical or panoramic
fixed bridge	periapical or panoramic	panoramic, tomographic, or CT*
overdenture	panoramic	lateral cephalogram or CT*
*radiographic guide may be required		

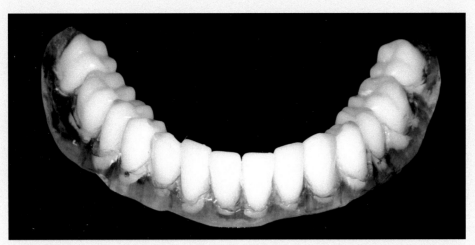

Fig 3-24 Radiologic guide with tooth position determined by the diagnostic waxup and processed with radioopaque teeth and acrylic resin.

patient. Once this is done, the dentist will then ask the implant surgeon for a consultation regarding the plan. The surgeon may require further diagnostic images and may consult with a radiologist. At this stage, the need for a radiographic guide and its design should be discussed. Recent guidelines have been published on the use of diagnostic imaging for implant dentistry. Each patient should be assessed individually with a view to obtaining essential diagnostic images, but with the minimum possible radiation exposure.

Construction of radiological guide

A resin guide can serve two purposes: to demonstrate the position of the definitive restorations on a radiograph, and as a surgical guide to aid the surgeon in placing the implant in the correct position at the time of surgery. It is usually possible to use one guide for both purposes. This type of guide may be used with all types of radiography (Fig 3-24).

The radiological guide is constructed as follows:
- working casts are made from accurate impressions of the teeth
- a diagnostic waxup of the definitive restoration is completed to the correct contours and occlusal plane. If the patient has a satisfactory removable partial or complete denture, this may be duplicated and used as a guide
- the diagnostic waxup is duplicated using radio-opaque resin teeth. The denture base is processed with clear acrylic resin to provide stability for the guide on neighboring teeth or soft tissue
- for screw-retained restorations, it is helpful to drill a hole through the lingual/occlusal site on the tooth where the final screw should emerge.

The patient is instructed to arrive at the dental office just before the radiograph is taken and the guide inserted. After the radiograph is taken, the guide can be removed by the patient and returned to the dental office in case the radiograph will need to be repeated.

Once the radiological analysis has been completed and the final selection of the size and the position of the implant ascertained, the guide may be converted for surgical use. This will aid the surgeon when the implants are placed at the time of stage one surgery.

Implant Treatment Planning

Study casts

The use of mounted study casts is an essential component in the formulation of a treatment plan. This is the best method to ensure that vital information is available before treatment begins. From an analysis of the casts it is possible to assess the potential sites for implant placement. The following features should be considered:

- remaining dentition—alignment, overeruption, size and shape of teeth
- mesiodistal and buccolingual width of edentulous ridge
- vertical height from edentulous ridge to occlusal plane
- static and dynamic occlusal relationships between the mandible and the maxilla.

Diagnostic waxup

The diagnostic waxup is the key to the planning and execution of implant restorations (Fig 4-1). The radiographic guide, surgical guide, and provisional and definitive restorations are based on the waxup. It is invaluable as a communication tool between the patient, restorative dentist, laboratory technician, and surgeon.

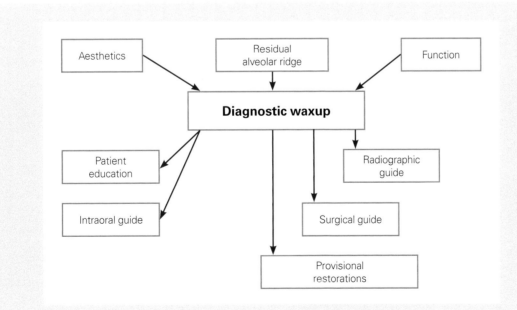

Fig 4-1 Proper use of the diagnostic waxup is the key to optimizing the entire treatment.

A fully contoured diagnostic waxup is carried out on casts mounted on a semi-adjustable articulator (Fig 4-2). In the case of a single missing tooth, the diagnostic waxup is often a simple procedure, but it may become difficult where there are several missing teeth or in cases of inadequate space distribution, asymmetry, or occlusal problems. The waxup allows the implant team to assess the mesiodistal, buccolingual, and interocclusal distances. It allows an initial assessment of the width and number of implants that will be required. The waxup may be demonstrated to the patient in order to highlight specific problems.

Where significant aesthetic changes are planned, it is often helpful to make a light vacuum-formed plastic guide based on the waxup. This guide can be used intraorally with quick-setting resin to show the patient what they might expect at the end of treatment (Fig 4-3). It is worth spending time at the diagnostic waxup stage to make sure that the best possible restoration is planned and that the patient is fully informed. Once finalized, the diagnostic waxup allows the technician to construct radiographic and surgical guides that will aid the surgeon in placing the implants.

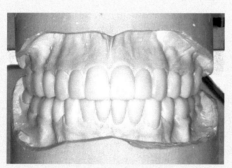 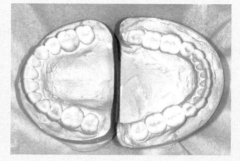

Fig 4-2 A fully contoured diagnostic waxup.

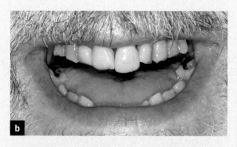

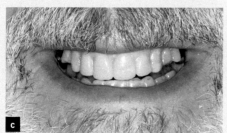

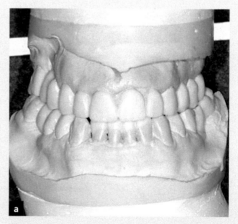

Fig 4-3 (a–c) Resin replica of diagnostic waxup placed over the existing teeth to illustrate the position and contour of planned restorations.

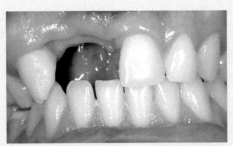

Fig 4-4 Bone deficiency related to missing anterior teeth.

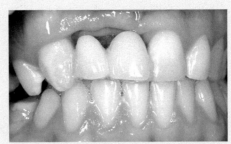

Fig 4-5 Acrylic template constructed from the diagnostic waxup demonstrating the extent of tissue deficiency and assisting the surgeon in planning any augmentation procedures.

It is essential for the dentist to fully assess the amount of tissue that is missing when implants are being considered (Fig 4-4). A diagnostic waxup will show any bony deficiencies in the sites of the planned implants and, hence, warn the surgeon that augmentation procedures may be required, either before or at the time of surgery. An acrylic template can be constructed from the diagnostic waxup transferred to the mouth to illustrate—both to patient and surgeon—the final tooth position relative to the existing supporting tissue (Fig 4-5).

Number of implants

The number of implants that are required for any given space must be determined at the diagnostic stage of treatment. The main factors are:

- number of teeth being replaced
- mesiodistal length of edentulous space—how many implants can be accommodated
- aesthetic requirements—natural spacing of teeth, soft tissue contours
- location in the arch—posterior teeth require more support than anterior teeth
- type of opposing dentition—removable denture versus teeth or fixed prosthesis
- parafunction—excessive force may indicate the use of more implants.

When planning the number of implants to support multiple replacement teeth, it is useful to consider all aspects of the edentulous space. As with conventional bridgework, aesthetic and functional factors make each case unique, and guidelines are based more on clinical experience than solid evidence.

It is not always necessary, or even desirable, to place one implant for each missing tooth (Fig 4-6). In many instances, one implant may be used to support two teeth, or two implants may support three teeth (Fig 4-7). Many surgeons believe that it is more difficult to reconstruct an interdental papilla

55

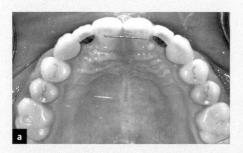

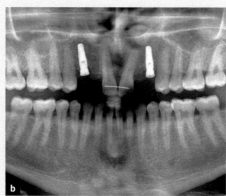

Fig 4-6 (a and b) Cantilevered restoration of upper lateral incisors from implants in the canine sites.

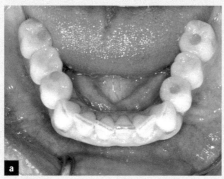

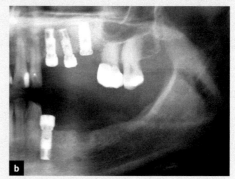

Fig 4-7 Example of two implants supporting a three-unit restoration on each side of the mandible (a) where machanical, occlusal and biological factors are favorable. When there is an unfavorable crown/implant ratio, or bone quality is reduced, it is preferable to place an implant for each tooth to be replaced (b).

between two adjacent implant-supported teeth than between an implant-supported tooth and a cantilevered pontic. This means that cantilevered restorations may give better results where aesthetic demands are high. However, cantilevered pontics placed posteriorly in the dental arch will be subject to high occlusal loads and are more likely to fail. An opposing natural dentition—especially with any degree of parafunction—will exert greater force on restorations than a removable denture and would be an indication for more implant support. In general, molar teeth should be replaced with an implant for each missing unit. Anteriorly, there is more scope for the use of cantilevered or fixed-bridge designs.

For the restoration of small edentulous spaces (one to three missing teeth), it is critical to verify that there is adequate mesiodistal space for replacement teeth and implants. First, determine if there is the correct mesiodistal space to provide the replacement teeth. In the aesthetic zone, symmetry of the teeth is very important: where a tooth (or teeth) is missing; then the best guide for space required is to measure the size of the contralateral tooth (or teeth). Where teeth are missing bilaterally, tables of standard tooth sizes can be used as a guide for the replacement teeth (Table 4-1).

Table 4-1 Approximate mesiodistal diameter of teeth (mm).

	Central incisor	Lateral incisor	Canine	First premolar	Second premolar	First molar	Second molar
Maxilla	9	6.5	9	7	7	10.5	10
Mandible	5.5	6	7	7	7	11	10.5

Difficulties arise where the space is too large or too small for the replacement tooth. The diagnostic waxup will reveal potential problems with restorations in this situation, including loss of symmetry, residual spaces, food packing, and poor interproximal contacts (Fig 4-8). These issues must be addressed before implant treatment begins; extractions, orthodontic therapy, or other restorations may be required to achieve adequate space for replacement teeth.

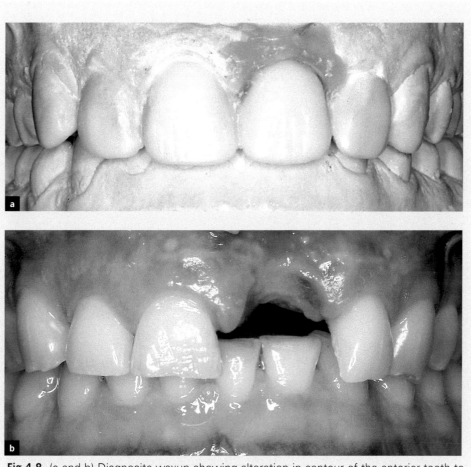

Fig 4-8 (a and b) Diagnositc waxup showing alteration in contour of the anterior teeth to compensate for the larger space present in the upper-left central incisor site.

Once it is established that adequate space is available for tooth replacement, clinical and radiographic measurements are used to determine if sufficient space exists for the implant(s), so that it/they can be surrounded on all sides by at least 1 mm of bone (Fig 4-9). Each implant will require at least 1 mm of bone on either side, plus 0.25 mm to avoid contact with the adjacent periodontal ligament, i.e.:

width of space ≥ width of implant + 2.5 mm

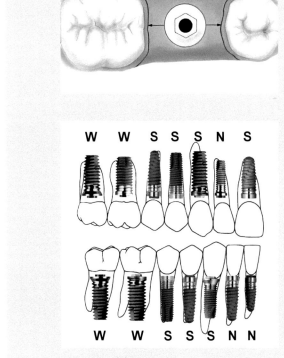

Fig 4-9 Ideal position of implant relative to the adjacent teeth.

Fig 4-10 Implants are selected to best restore the tooth they are replacing (W = wide diameter; S = standard diameter; N = narrow diameter). Anteriorly, the space available for an implant may be limited and so a tapered design may be used (e.g., the lower central incisor shown above). Posteriorly, the teeth are usually larger than the implants used to replace them.

So for an implant 4.1 mm in diameter, a minimum mesiodistal space of 6.6 mm is required, but 7–8 mm would be preferred. For more than one implant, the space equation needs to be multiplied by the number of implants being used. Ideally, at least 7 mm of mesiodistal space should be allowed for each standard platform implant to be placed. In the case of mandibular incisors and maxillary lateral incisors, there is often less than 7 mm of mesiodistal space available, and so a smaller implant may be used (Fig 4-10). For the replacement of molar teeth, there will generally be more than 7mm of space for the implant, so a larger implant may be used. It is important not to place implants too close together, as it difficult to restore the embrasure spaces adequately. This results in gingival inflammation, poor aesthetics, and difficulty with cleaning.

It has been suggested that a molar should be replaced using two implants instead of one. Placement of two standard implants in a molar site will distribute occlusal forces more evenly than one, and more closely matches the emergence profile of the natural tooth (Fig 4-11). However, two implants placed very close together are difficult to restore and may result in bone loss between them (Fig 4-12). Inability to clean adequately between the implants may lead to gingival inflammation.

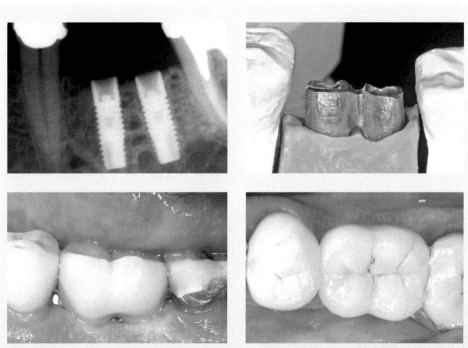

Fig 4-11 Two implants used to support a molar restoration. Note the small space between the abutment and tissue, which leads to difficulty in cleaning the furcation area.

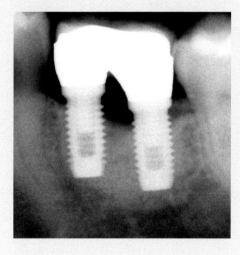

Fig 4-12 Radiograph showing interproximal bone loss between two implants supporting a single tooth.

Position of implants

Ideally, implants should be oriented along the long axis of the tooth that is being replaced to ensure axial loading and to avoid complications with the restorative procedures. The position of the implant head in three dimensions is critical to the achievement of the final aesthetic result (Fig 4-13).

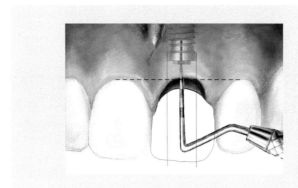

Fig 4-13 Diagram of implant oriented along the axis of the tooth it is replacing and placed 2–3 mm apical to the cementoenamel junction of the adjacent teeth.

The implant should be centered mesiodistally in the replacement tooth space to avoid encroaching on embrasures and marginal gingiva. If the implant is too close to the adjacent teeth or other implants it will be difficult to achieve the best emergence profile or gingival health (Fig 4-14).

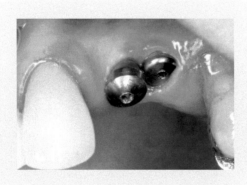

Fig 4-14 Implants placed too close together can be impossible to restore adequately. It may be necessary to leave one implant unused if it cannot be removed without damaging the other implant.

The implant should be positioned within the occlusal outline of the replacement tooth to create the optimum emergence profile. This minimizes the possibility of abnormally shaped prostheses, leading to problems with gingival health, poor aesthetics, and speech difficulties (Fig 4-15).

Vertically, the implant should be above bone level, but apical enough to create the proper emergence profile. Generally, the implant head should be 2–3 mm apical to the cementoenamel junction

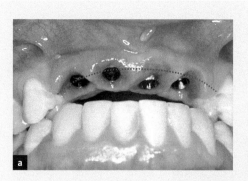
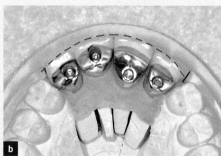
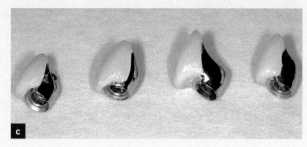

Fig 4-15 An example of implants placed too far palatally, leading to abnormally-shaped restorations that are difficult to maintain.

of the adjacent teeth. The implant position should maintain the gingival health and allow appropriate embrasure spaces for cleaning and aesthetics. Implants placed too far apically will lead to crown–root ratios that are aesthetically and biomechanically challenging (Fig 4-16). Implants placed superficially make it difficult to achieve a good emergence profile on the restoration (Fig 4-17).

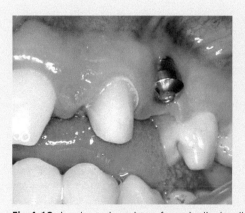
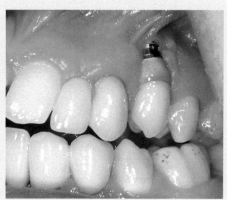

Fig 4-16 Implant placed too far apically, leading to an unaesthetic restoration with an unfavorable crown–implant ratio.

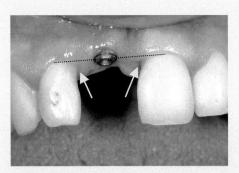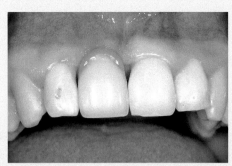

Fig 4-17 Implant placed too superficially, leading to difficulty in creating an aesthetic restoration. The dotted line shows the implant to be too superficial—at the CEJ level of the neighboring teeth—and the yellow arrows show loss of interdental papillae. Pink-colored porcelain
is attempting to compensate for the difficult emergence profile due to implant placement.

The distance from the alveolar ridge to the incisal edge of the opposing teeth is an important
measurement. The success of the final restoration will depend upon whether there is enough space
available to accommodate all the necessary components and the final restoration (Fig 4-18). As a
guide, the minimum vertical space that is required is dependent upon the type of abutment connector
and restoration that is used, and can vary from 4.5 to 7.5 mm.

Studies by Tarnow and colleagues have demonstrated that the thickness of mucosa covering the
bone between two implants is 2–4 mm (Fig 4-19). Furthermore, an interimplant distance of at least
3 mm will be more likely to maintain the soft tissues. Note that the tissue height between adjacent
implants is approximately 2 mm less than occurs between natural adjacent teeth. Great care should
be taken when placing adjacent implants in the aesthetic zone.

The placement should allow the restorative dentist to have good access to any screw exit locations and good restorative access.

Selection of implants

Today, implants are manufactured in a variety of different shapes, sizes, and surface treatments, making implant selection more complex. There are a number of factors that influence implant selection
for an individual case (see Table 4-2).

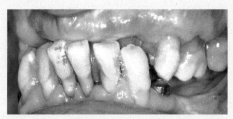

Fig 4-18 Insufficent vertical space for restoration of the implant in the lower-left premolar region.

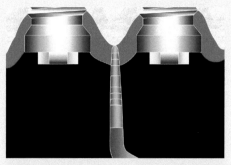

Fig 4-19 The papilla between two adjacent implants is 2–4 mm. (Reproduced from Tarnow et al 2003 with permission from the American Academy of Periodontology).

Table 4-2 Some of the factors that influence implant selection.

Implant site	Influences selection of
size of the tooth that is being replaced	implant surface area
bone quality	implant surface
available bone height	implant length
alveolar ridge width	implant diameter
initial implant stability	implant size and thread design
abutment screw stress	implant diameter
emergence profile of the restoration	restorative platform

Implant length

The longer the implant, the greater the surface that is available for bone-to-implant contact. Generally, the aim is to place the longest fixture that is clinically and radiographically possible. Bicortical fixation is desirable, though not essential, in order to give good initial fixation of the implant when it is inserted. Standard implants are generally available from 7–18 mm in length. As an implant increases in length by 3 mm, there is an increase of bone-to-implant contact of approximately 20%.

Implant diameter

When implants are placed, each one should be surrounded by at least 1 mm of bone so that stability and osseointegration are not compromised (Fig 4-20).

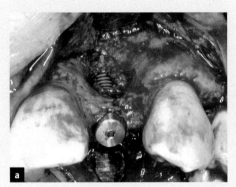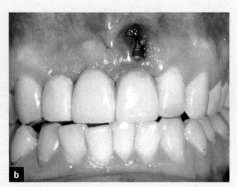

Fig 4-20 (a) Fenestration of buccal plate of bone, showing incomplete encasement of the implant, (b) failed restoration due to fenestration of the implant.

The width of alveolar bone is difficult to determine precisely from clinical examination or study casts alone. If it is thought that there is sufficient bone for implants, the diameter of implant may be chosen at the time of surgery, when the alveolar bone is visible. When clinical examination suggests that alveolar bone may be limited, cross-sectional radiographs, in combination with radiographic guides, may be necessary to measure the width and depth of bone available for implant placement.

Ideally, dental implants would be the same size as the teeth they replace, though this is rarely the case. In order to achieve a good emergence profile and reduce the risk of fracture, it is preferable to place an implant that approaches the size of the missing tooth (Fig 4-21). Dental implants are now made in a variety of diameters, which are comparable to average tooth diameters (Fig 4-22).

Standard implants

There is no direct relationship between the dimensions of a "standard" implant (approximately 4 mm) and a tooth. In many cases, these implants have a smaller diameter than the teeth they are replacing. This mismatch between implant and tooth dimension may cause difficulties with the emergence profile and aesthetics of the final restoration. Standard implants are generally a compromise between the aesthetic demands of the prosthesis and the amount of bone and space available for implant placement.

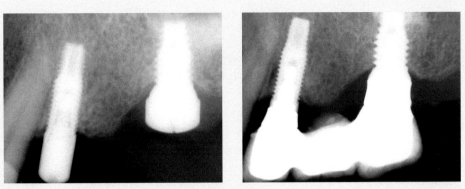

Fig 4-21 Radiographs showing different-sized implants for the replacement of teeth of different sizes.

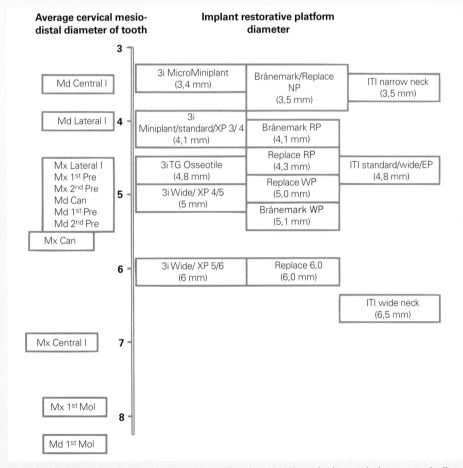

Fig 4-22 Diagram showing the diameters of various implant designs relative to mesiodistal tooth width.

Implants with narrow diameters

There are situations where the space for replacing a tooth is limited, such as the lower incisors and upper maxillary lateral incisors (Fig 4-23). It is also difficult to achieve an appropriate emergence profile for a narrow tooth on a wider implant body. In these situations, it is often helpful to use an implant with a narrow restorative platform. However, the restorative components for narrow implants differ from those needed for other implants.

A thin alveolar ridge may be another indication for narrow-bodied implants, as it may alleviate the necessity for additional surgical procedures such as ridge augmentation, bone grafting, or guided tissue regeneration. As a rough guide, narrow implants can be used where there is less than 7 mm of mesiodistal space and where the ridge is less than 6 mm wide.

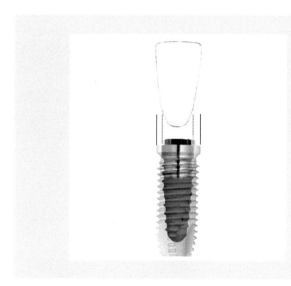

Fig 4-23 For smaller-diameter teeth, such as mandibular incisors, it is only possible to achieve a good emergence profile for the restoration by using a narrow-platform implant (dotted line). The width of a standard-diameter implant is shown for comparison (solid line).

The clinical success of narrow implants is not as well documented as that of standard implants. It should be recognized that narrow implants have less bone-contact area and smaller restorative components than standard implants, and may be more prone to failure. Narrow implants should not generally be used where a larger implant could be placed successfully.

Implants with wide diameters

Wide-diameter implants offer several advantages over standard implants. Care must be taken by the surgeon, when placing these implants, that sufficient bone is available on all sides of the fixture. In areas where the quality of bone is poor, such as the maxillary and mandibular posterior regions, wide implants may engage the buccal and lingual cortical plates of bone. This allows the implant to resist any lateral movement and gives good initial stability during healing, which will enhance the ability of the implant to integrate.

Wide implants are particularly useful in immediate extraction sites as they occupy more space in the tooth socket. This brings more of the implant into contact with the bony walls of the socket, which will improve initial stability and require less bone regeneration around the implant during osseointegration (Fig 4-24). A wider diameter implant may also be used to replace a standard implant that has failed to integrate.

Wide-diameter implants are also desirable when the height of bone is limited and shorter implants must be placed; for example in the posterior maxilla or in the mandible over the inferior dental nerve. Wide-diameter implants have considerably greater surface area than standard implants (Fig 4-25). For example, a 6 mm x 10 mm implant has 61% more surface area than a 3.75 mm x 10 mm implant.

By taking full advantage of the bone that is available, a wide-diameter implant may avoid the necessity for more complex surgical procedures such as sinus grafting in the maxilla and nerve repositioning in the lower arch.

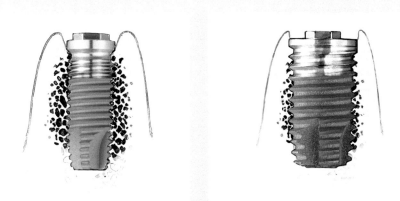

Fig 4-24 In a wide alveolar ridge, a standard diameter implant may engage mainly cancellous bone *(left)*, reducing initial stabilty of the implant. A wide-diameter implant may engage the cortex of the alveolar ridge *(right)*, resulting in greater initial stability.

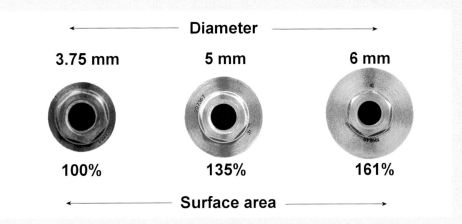

Fig 4-25 Diagram showing the increase in implant surface area as the diameter increases.

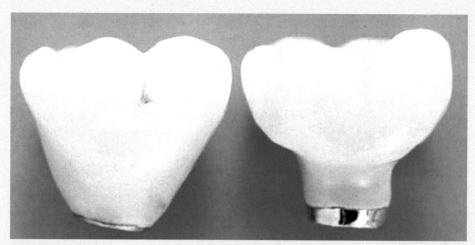

Fig 4-26 Photograph of molar crowns made on a 6 mm-diameter implant *(left)* compared to a 3.75 mm implant *(right)*. Note the more natural emergence profile of the restoration on the wider implant.

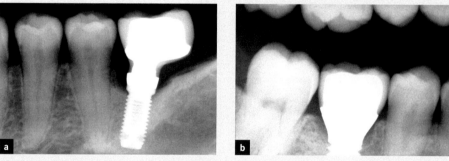

Fig 4-27 Mismatch of crown size to implant diameter leading to poor emergence profile and high stress on the implant assembly (a). A more ideal emergence profile of a crown placed on a wide-diameter implant makes for easier maintenance and better stress distribution (b).

Increasing the implant diameter also significantly expands the seating surface area of the implant. In molar teeth, wide-diameter implants facilitate a more natural emergence profile than standard implants (Fig 4-26). In addition, wider implants provide a greater load-bearing area between the implant and the restoration or the abutment, thereby reducing stress on the retaining screw (Fig 4-27).

Tapered implants

A narrow or concave alveolar ridge is sometimes present where there is insufficient bone to place a parallel-sided implant of the required diameter. To overcome this problem, implants have been developed that have a tapering body and a wider restorative platform (Fig 4-28). This design combines the advantages of good stability and acceptable emergence profile. Tapered implants may also be useful in circumstances where a cylindrical implant might impinge on the periodontal ligament if there is

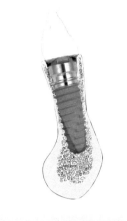

Fig 4-28 Diagram illustrating where a tapered implant may be used in a narrow alveolar ridge without perforating the cortical plate of bone.

some convergence of adjacent roots. These types of implants may, therefore, provide good aesthetic results in cases where narrower implant bodies are the only option. Tapered implants may be especially useful for immediate or early replacement following tooth extraction (Fig 4-29). However, this approach is surgically technique sensitive and unpredictable in the aesthetic zone.

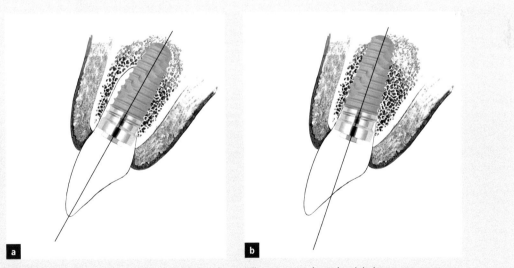

Fig 4-29 An implant may be used in an immediate extraction site (a); however, a space results between the implant and the bony socket. In order to minimize this, and provide improved stability, the angulation of a tapered implant may be changed to engage the cortical plate with less risk of perforation (b). In addition, the implant stability can be enhanced by engaging the bone apical to the extraction socket.

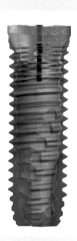

Fig 4-30 Extended platform implant superimposed on a standard implant of the same platform diameter (blue). The tapered platform and tapered body are useful in creating the correct emergence profile where the alveolar ridge is too narrow to place a standard implant.

Both parallel-sided and tapered implants are available with an extended restorative platform. This design allows for a normal emergence profile to be achieved, even when the local anatomy only permits a narrow implant to be placed (Fig 4-30). The extended restorative platform also provides better stability for the prosthesis and minimizes the potential for screw loosening, compared to a standard platform.

Emergence profile

A more natural emergence profile is achievable wherever it is possible to match the implant size to the cross-section of the tooth being replaced. Ideally, the implant diameter should be slightly less than the diameter of the tooth, as measured at the cementoenamel junction. With approximately the same dimensions as the replacement tooth, temporary healing abutments of various diameters have been developed to support the soft tissues during healing. The healing abutment is placed on the implant at the second-stage surgery and remains until a provisional or definitive restoration is in place. Healing abutments are placed on non-submerged implants at the time of implant placement.

A provisional restoration may also be used to develop and maintain the ideal emergence profile for a restoration. A carefully contoured and polished provisional crown will support the soft tissues and encourage healing after second-stage surgery is performed, or in combination with tissue augmentation (Fig 4-31).

External versus internal connection

Abutments either attach to a hexagon on the top of the implant (external connection) or fit into the implant itself (internal connection) (Fig 4-32). Both types of implant have been used successfully and neither design appears to have a clear clinical advantage.

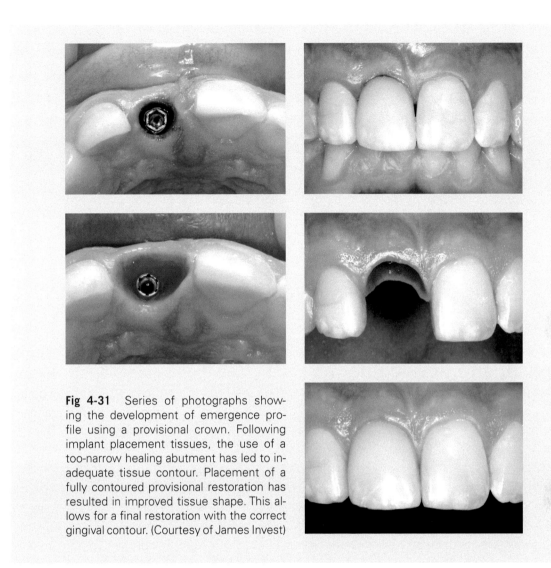

Fig 4-31 Series of photographs showing the development of emergence profile using a provisional crown. Following implant placement tissues, the use of a too-narrow healing abutment has led to inadequate tissue contour. Placement of a fully contoured provisional restoration has resulted in improved tissue shape. This allows for a final restoration with the correct gingival contour. (Courtesy of James Invest)

From a restorative point of view, because similar abutments are available for internal and external connection implants, the same range of restorations may be fabricated. Many practitioners find it easier to determine whether components are correctly seated in an internal connection, which improves the predictability of impression taking and abutment placement. In theory, the stronger internal connection leads to less stress concentration at the crestal bone, though it is not clear if this is clinically significant.

The internal surface of some implants may also incorporate a machined 8° tapered surface, known as a Morse taper. This feature provides a stable connection between the implant and abutment and minimizes the gap between the two components.

It would appear that the correct placement of the dental implant is more important than the type of connection in determining the success of the final restoration.

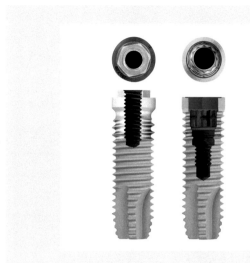

Fig 4-32 Examples of dental implants with external *(left)* and internal *(right)* abutment connections.

Surgical site development

The assessment of supporting tissues is a critical part of implant treatment planning. Often there is significant loss of supporting structures at an implant site. The causes of tooth loss, such as trauma or periodontal disease, will themselves result in bone resorption. Even so-called atraumatic extraction of teeth will end with alveolar resorption, since alveolar bone exists to support the teeth. Alveolar resorption is progressive, and patients may present for implants many years after loss of their teeth and alveolar bone.

At assessment, the restorative dentist must picture the ideal replacement for the missing tooth or teeth. An existing fixed or removable denture is often helpful in this regard. If this is not available, a diagnostic waxup must be made. Any vertical or horizontal space between the replacement teeth and the residual alveolar ridge (e.g, the pink "gum" on a removable denture) will have to be masked in the final restoration (Fig 4-33).

For example, if there is a 3 mm vertical loss of alveolar bone, the replacement teeth will have to be 3 mm longer than the ideal length. In patients with a low lip line, or in areas that are not aesthetically critical, this may be acceptable (Fig 4-34); however, in many cases such a result is unacceptable aesthetically and may also result in unfavorable crown–implant ratios (Fig 4-35).

Similarly, a horizontal discrepancy between the position of the implant site (i.e. the alveolar bone) and the final restoration may cause aesthetic difficulties or mechanical failure of implant components.

A common limitation to implant placement, particularly in the anterior part of the mandible, is a thin residual alveolar ridge. This situation may be deceptive because the vertical discrepancy between restoration and bone seems small, but, in fact, the alveolar ridge is too thin for implants. At implant placement, the surgeon will "flatten" the narrow ridge ("ramp down") until a wider implant site is

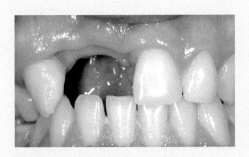
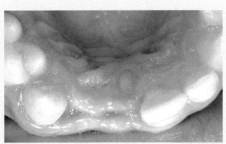
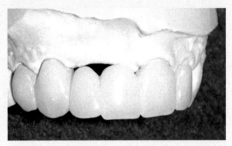

Fig 4-33 Extraction of teeth generally results in vertical and horizontal hard and soft tissue defects. The amount of tissue replacement required can be visualized by construction of a temporary restoration.

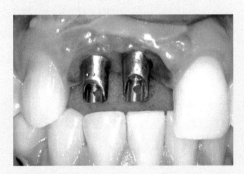
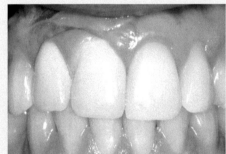
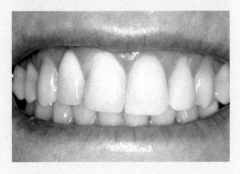

Fig 4-34 A smaller anterior tissue defect can be masked using pink-colored porcelain with a favorable lip line.

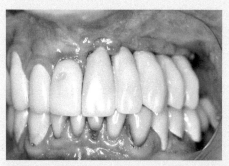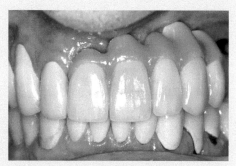

Fig 4-35 Extensive tissue deficiency resulting in elongated and angulated provisional crowns. Use of pink porcelain in the definitive restoration to mask the tissue defect may improve the appearance of the crowns.

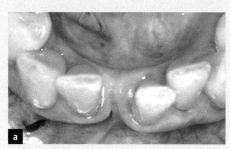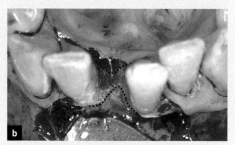

Fig 4-36 Typical soft tissue (a) and hard tissue (b) defects in the anterior mandible.

reached, resulting in a more apically placed implant and a significant vertical discrepancy. Localized bone defects may also lead to fenestration or dehiscence of the implant during placement and hence poorer conditions for healing (Fig 4-36).

In order to optimize implant and restorative success, it is often advisable or essential to enlarge the residual ridge before or during implant placement. Ridge augmentation should be considered whenever the restorative dentist has determined that an acceptable aesthetic or functional result cannot be achieved prosthetically. The details of these procedures are outside the scope of this book, but several accounts have been published (Esposito et al, 2006). However, the restorative dentist should recognize that augmentation procedures add to the cost and usually the time taken to complete implant restorations. The restorative dentist must work closely with the implant surgeon to understand the potential and limitations of alveolar ridge augmentation. Overall, little robust clinical data exist to support one technique over another and patients should be advised that an acceptable result cannot be guaranteed.

Larger deficiencies in the alveolar ridge are more difficult to correct than small defects and generally have less predictable success. Vertical defects are more challenging than horizontal bone loss, and they may not be resolved to the patient's, or dentist's, satisfaction. Prevention of bone loss is preferable to repair, and it is often advantageous to provide immediate or early implant placement following tooth loss. Alternatively, the surgeon may elect to place a graft material in the extraction socket to reduce the potential for resorption, and then place the implant several weeks or months later.

Hard tissue grafting

Where the residual alveolar ridge itself is inadequate for implant placement, augmentation of the bone must be considered (Fig 4-37). Autogenous bone is the "gold standard" for bone grafting, since it contains living cells with osteogenic potential (Fig 4-38). This is bone that is taken from another site in the same patient. However, it is difficult to harvest sufficient bone from oral sites to graft sizeable bone defects. Autogenous bone may be mixed with another grafting material to augment larger deficiencies. There is a wide range of commercially available graft materials, of which the most common are alloplastic materials, xenografts, and allografts.

Alloplastic materials are synthetic and available in a variety of formats, though the porous particulate type is most frequently used for implant surgery. These materials are mostly based on calcium phosphate, calcium sulfate, or bioactive glass (ceramic). Though considered to be osteoconductive, facilitating bone formation, each alloplast has somewhat different characteristics in terms of hardness and its rate of replacement by bone.

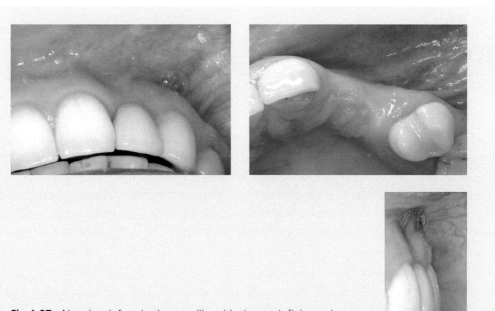

Fig 4-37 Alveolar defect in the maxilla with tissue deficiency in both the horizontal and vertical aspects.

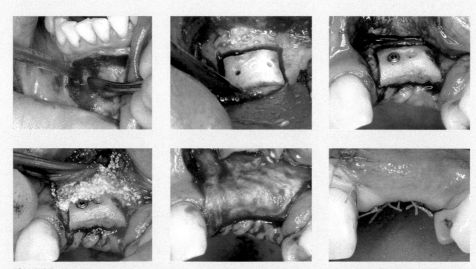

Fig 4-38 Placement of autogenous bone graft in the defect shown in Fig 4-37. Bone is harvested from the chin, fixed over the defect with screws, covered with particulate graft and a membrane, and sutured. (Courtesy of Dr. P.J. Byrne)

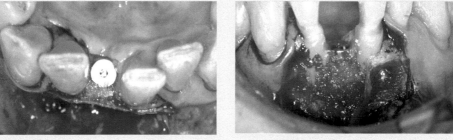

Fig 4-39 Particulate allograft material used to augment the bone surrounding a mandibular implant.

These characteristics must be borne in mind when planning subsequent implant placement, especially if the implant is to be placed within the grafted area. Xenografts based on deproteinized bovine bone are also used for alveolar augmentation and to mix with autogenous bone (Fig 4-39). The osteoconductive matrix is gradually replaced by bone, though it is difficult to quantify how much loss of graft volume occurs in the process.

Allograft bone enjoys some popularity as an augmentation material, though it is controversial because it is derived from human cadavers. The bone is freeze-dried and may, additionally, be demineralized, but it retains bioactive growth factors such as the bone morphogenetic proteins (BMPs). Some studies have demonstrated that bone allografts are osteoinductive, though this is not always predictable.

Particulate grafts are most appropriate for filling small and well-defined (multi-walled) bony defects. However, increasing the height or width of the alveolar ridge generally requires an onlay graft, consisting of a block of autogenous bone. The oral donor sites (chin, ramus) have limited potential and are associated with significant morbidity. Substantial onlay grafts must be harvested from large bones, such as the hip, which necessitates hospitalization, and the procedure has potential complications. Obviously, the patient must be fully aware of the risks and benefits of these procedures, and the restorative dentist should be clear about what can be achieved through their use.

Soft tissue grafting

In some instances there is sufficient alveolar bone to place dental implants in a good position to support the final restoration, but a tissue deficiency still remains. This deficiency in the tissue may be horizontal or vertical and would lead to aesthetic, phonetic, or maintenance problems with the restoration. A common example of tissue deficiency is the "black triangle," which is seen between teeth where the normal gingival is missing (Fig 4-40a). Another example is the root eminences, which are normally present with natural teeth, but very difficult to maintain over implants (Fig 4-40b).

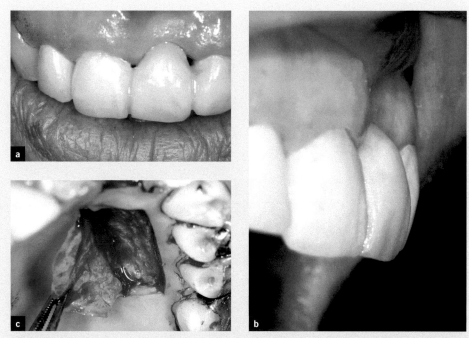

Fig 4-40 (a) Loss of gingival tissue leading to the formation of "black triangles", (b) increased pontic length, and loss of facial contour. (c) Harvesting of a connective tissue graft from the palate. (Courtesy of Dr. J. Lack)

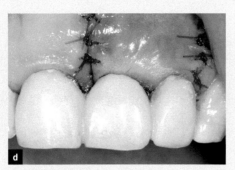
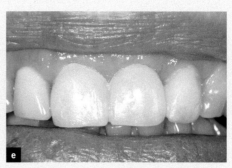

Fig 4-40 (d) Graft sutured into position with a provisional restoration, (e) healed graft ready for placement of a dental implant. (Courtesy of Dr. J. Lack)

Additional soft tissue around an implant may resolve an aesthetic or functional difficulty. The tissue may be augmented by the use of a subepithelial connective tissue graft. In this procedure, a block of connective tissue is harvested from the palate (Fig 4-40c) and then placed under the mucosa where it is needed to add bulk to the residual alveolar ridge (Fig 4-40d). The tissue may be grafted as a separate procedure before implant placement, or at the same time as implant placement. At any rate, it will take several months for the grafted site to attain its final contour (Fig 4-40e). Any restoration related to the grafted site—such as the alveolar ridge crest—must be delayed until healing of the graft has occurred.

It can be very challenging to replace the soft tissue around dental implants—for example, if there is no inter-implant strut of bone to support a gingival papilla—since the underlying bone support is different to that which exists around teeth (Figs 4-41, 4-42).

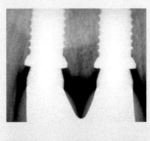
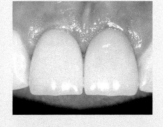

Fig 4-41 Good inter-implant bone support on platform-switched restorations, resulting in the maintenance of the interdental papilla and soft tissue contour.

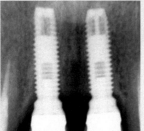
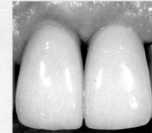

Fig 4-42 Loss of inter-implant supporting bone resulting in the absence of an interdental papilla (courtesy of Dr. R. Cochetto).

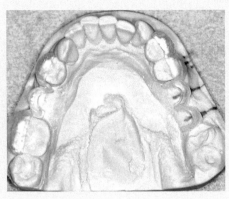

Fig 4-43 Implant surgical guide for the replacement of missing mandibular teeth. This guide is tooth-borne so as not to interfere with soft tissue flaps, and it allows access for osteotomy preparation on its lingual side.

Surgical guide construction

The purpose of a surgical guide is to allow the surgeon to place the implants in the best possible position (Fig 4-43). The guide should be based on a diagnostic waxup of the missing tooth or teeth. To facilitate implant placement, the guide should:

- show the replacement tooth position and inclination
- show the incisal edge/buccal cusp and cementoenamel junction of the replacement tooth
- indicate the location of the cingulum or central fossa
- allow access to the surgical site so the implant will be placed in the correct alignment
- not alter the required flap design
- be easily placed and stable at the time of surgery.

The surgical guide is made from cast that has a diagnostic waxup of the missing teeth. This waxup should be checked by the restorative dentist and used for the radiologic guide, where indicated. Once approved, the waxup should be returned to the laboratory for construction of the surgical guide. There are variations in the design of surgical guides, depending on the operator and the number of missing teeth. Guides are constructed of clear acrylic resin and may include metal tubes to aid the surgeon in preparing the implant sites. Many surgeons prefer greater flexibility for implant placement. Common methods for guide construction include the following:

- the facial surfaces of the teeth that are being replaced should be reproduced according to the diagnostic waxup
- the lingual/buccal surfaces of the replacement teeth should be cut away, leaving intact the interproximal areas adjacent to the edentulous space. This can then be used to guide the surgeon when the implants are being placed (Fig 4-44)

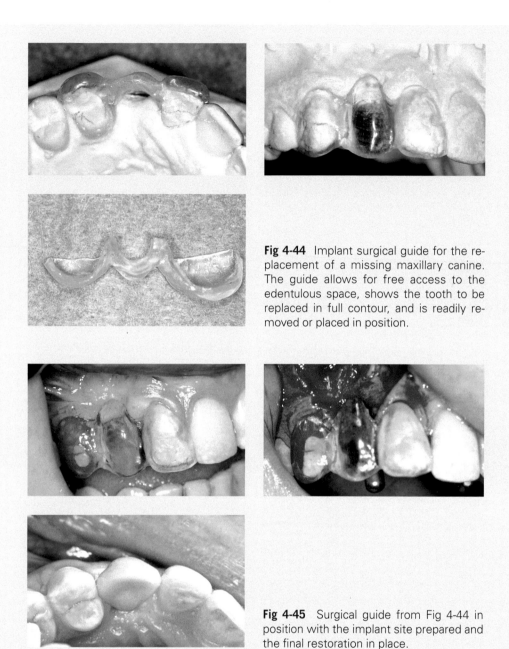

Fig 4-44 Implant surgical guide for the replacement of a missing maxillary canine. The guide allows for free access to the edentulous space, shows the tooth to be replaced in full contour, and is readily removed or placed in position.

Fig 4-45 Surgical guide from Fig 4-44 in position with the implant site prepared and the final restoration in place.

- the incisogingival (or occlusogingival) height of the replacement teeth is clearly shown on the guide, so that the surgeon is able to place the implant 2–3 mm below this mark. This will allow the final restoration to emerge out of the tissue and create an aesthetic restoration (Fig 4-45)
- the guide must be stable on the cast and in the mouth. This is achieved by ensuring that the acrylic overlays the incisal/occlusal surfaces of the remaining teeth

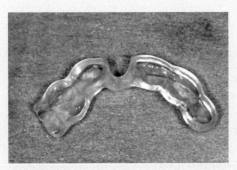
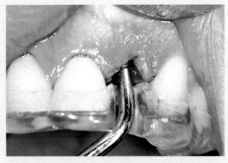

Fig 4-46 Facial access provided in the surgical guide. This design gives excellent visual access for placing implants.

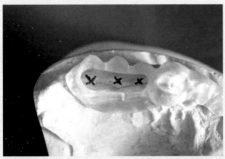
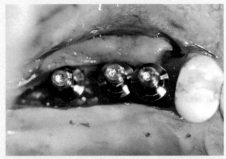

Fig 4-47 Trough design of surgical guide, allowing leeway in the placement of implants; however, it may result in implants that are too close to one another.

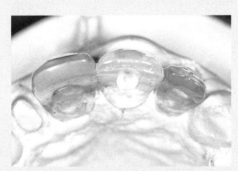
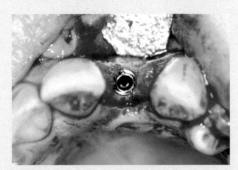

Fig 4-48 Full-contour, palatally approaching surgical guide, allowing accurate placement of an implant.

- the guide may be shortened in height, particularly in the posterior region of the mouth, in order to allow access for drilling
- there are many variations in guide design, depending on the implant site and degree of access and visibility. Some of these are shown in (Figs 4-46–4-49). The surgeon will have his/her own preference.

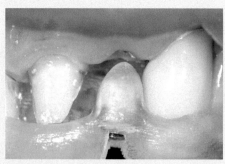 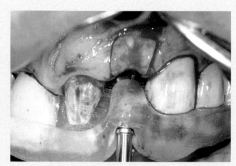

Fig 4-49 Computer-generated guides from a CT scan. Metal tube for drilling allows for complete control of implant alignment.

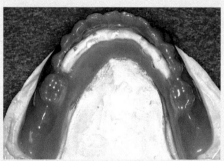 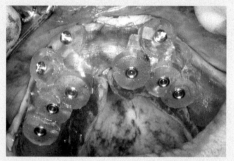

Fig 4-50 Soft tissue-borne surgical guide for implant placement in the anterior mandible. The guide should cover enough surface area to provide stability, yet allow for drilling access.

Fig 4-51 Surgical guide (with drilling tubes) screwed directly onto the maxilla for complete stability.

Where there are few remaining teeth, it may not be possible to construct a stable guide that rests only on the teeth. In this case, the guide will have to be tissue-borne (Fig 4-50). It is best to check the design of the guide with the surgeon to ensure that it will not interfere with the surgical site. It must be possible to position the guide accurately when the mucoperiosteal flaps have been raised for implant placement. In some cases this will entail fixation of the guide itself directly into the bone using small screws (Fig 4-51).

It is sometimes possible to modify the radiological guide and use it as a surgical guide. In this case, the radio-opaque teeth are ground to leave the facial surfaces intact. However, the design of the guide must allow for stable placement at the time of surgery and not interfere with the surgical site.

CHAPTER 5

Restorative Treatment Planning

Provisional restorations

During implant treatment, provisional restorations are generally required to maintain the edentulous space for both aesthetics and function. Depending on the number of teeth to be replaced, there are a number of options available. Initially, a removable prosthesis is less expensive than a fixed restoration, though this saving may be lost in the extra time that is required to carry out the necessary ongoing maintenance of the denture during implant therapy.

Adhesive fixed dental prostheses

Adhesive fixed dental prostheses may be cemented onto the adjacent teeth before, or at the time of, implant placement (Fig 5-1). The abutment teeth should not be prepared with guide planes, rest seats, or grooves, as would be the case if this type of fixed dental prosthesis was being used as a permanent restoration. A simple "Rochette" fixed dental prosthesis design with perforated retainers and a resin pontic may be used, as it will provide adequate retention for the healing period but is not too difficult to remove when required.

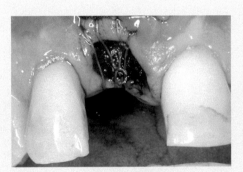
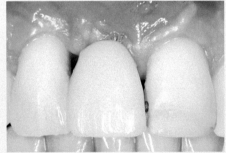
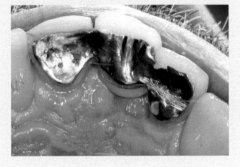

Fig 5-1 Extraction site of maxillary central incisor temporarily restored with an adhesive fixed dental prosthesis prior to implant placement.

The pontic should be adequately relieved in order to prevent any loading of the implant site (Fig 5-2). The pontic will usually need to be adjusted again after the second-stage surgery in order to accommodate the healing abutment. Alternatively, it may be advisable to adjust the healing abutment so that the adhesive fixed dental prosthesis can be replaced, but making sure that good healing of the soft tissue is not compromised (Fig 5-3).

Most patients prefer this type of restoration to a removable dental prosthesis, as it requires little maintenance during the healing phase. However, patients should be warned that there is a risk that the fixed dental prostheses will debond during the healing phase, and, if this should happen, they should return to the office for recementation. The saving in chairside time during the course of implant treatment, together with greater patient acceptance, makes this type of restoration generally preferable to a removable dental prosthesis.

Conventional fixed dental prostheses

If one or more of the teeth adjacent to the implant site is prepared for a crown (or if a crown is planned for the tooth), then a fixed dental prosthesis may be used as a provisional restoration. The fixed dental prosthesis may be a fixed-fixed, cantilever, or hybrid design (Fig 5-4). The conventional fixed dental prosthesis may be constructed before the implant surgery and fitted after the implant is placed (Fig 5-5). It has similar advantages to the adhesive fixed dental prosthesis and is less likely to become decemented. Like the adhesive fixed dental prosthesis, the occlusal forces should be controlled on a conventional fixed dental prosthesis to minimize flexure and the possibility of loosening.

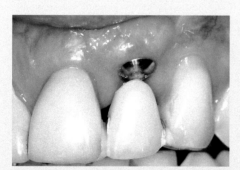

Fig 5-2 The pontic of the adhesive fixed dental prosthesis relieved to prevent loading of the implant and to facilitate cleaning by the patient.

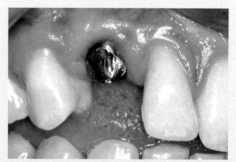

Fig 5-3 The healing abutment may also need to be adjusted to accommodate a provisional fixed restoration.

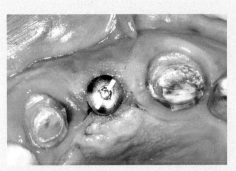
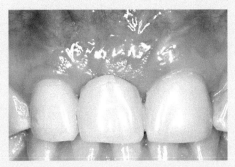

Fig 5-4 Simple acrylic resin provisional fixed dental prosthesis cemented onto the already-prepared adjacent teeth and replacing the maxillary right central incisor.

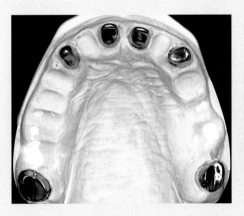
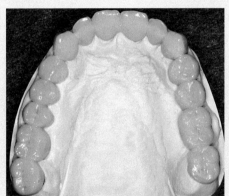

Fig 5-5 Complex provisional fixed dental prosthesis supported by non-precious metal copings to accommodate the placement of multiple implants. Copings are used to ensure the abutment teeth remain caries-free during treatment.

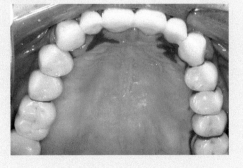

Removable dental prostheses

It may be possible to construct a removable prosthesis as a transitional restoration (Fig 5-6). If a removable prosthesis is used, it is essential that the implant site is not loaded between surgical stages. Tooth-borne dental prostheses, which will not load the implant site, are more suited than tissue-borne dental prostheses for use as transitional restorations. Similarly, maxillary prostheses, which are supported by the palate, are preferred over mandibular prostheses, which rest on the alveolar ridge only.

The following procedure should be followed:

- The prosthesis should, ideally, not be inserted for 10 to 14 days after stage-one surgery. After 1 week, the patient may wear the prosthesis for short periods only (a few hours), but not during function.
- The tissue-bearing area that is in contact with the implant site should be relieved to a depth of between 2 and 3 mm using a large acrylic bur in a straight handpiece.
- The prosthesis should be relined with a soft relining material (Visco-gel®, Dentsply DeTrey; Coe-Comfort, GC America Inc.; Sofreliner® Tokuyama Dental Corporation), following the manufacturer's instructions. Once the initial set has been achieved, the excess material is cut away using a sharp scalpel. It is essential that the tissue-bearing area has an adequate thickness of material to avoid overloading the implant site. If this is not achieved it will be necessary to remove both the reline material and additional acrylic from the prosthesis-bearing area, and then repeat the soft relining procedure.
- Soft relining materials deteriorate over a 4- to 6-week period and so will need to be replaced at least two or three times during the healing period.
- When a two-stage implant technique is used, healing abutments will be placed at the second-stage surgery. After this procedure, the dental prosthesis will need to be adjusted and relined again with the soft reliner material.

If the patient has an existing removable dental prosthesis this may be "converted" to an interim prosthesis for the healing period, provided that the stability and retention of the dental prosthesis are adequate. In addition, the dentist must ensure that sufficient thickness of soft reliner material may be accommodated. In order to adapt the dental prosthesis, the acrylic over the surgical site is generously relieved and relined as described above.

In the case of metal-based dental prostheses, it is often difficult to provide enough relief for reliner material in the thin metal. This will often be the case after the second-stage surgery, when healing abutments that protrude above the tissue height are placed. Perforation of the metal base might then occur with a resulting prosthesis that is difficult to maintain.

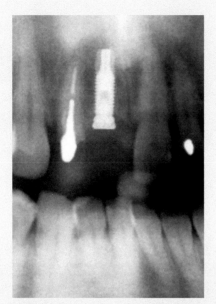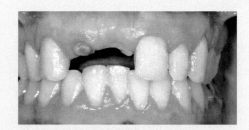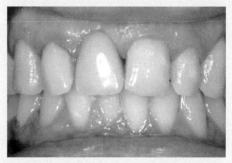

Fig 5-6 Removable dental prosthesis used as a provisional restoration following implant placement (central incisor) and extraction of the lateral incisor.

Provisional restoration of an implant

Placement of a provisional restoration of an implant may be necessary in order to allow healing of the soft tissue after surgery. The soft tissue may be supported and shaped by the contour of the provisional restoration leading to an improved aesthetic result. Provisionalization will allow the dentist to develop the optimum emergence profile while healing of the soft tissue takes place. Another advantage of the technique is that the patient can assess the aesthetic outcome of the final restoration at an early stage and appreciate any compromises that may be needed. There are a number of options that can be used to achieve this outcome:

- cement-retained restorations
- screw-retained restorations
- cement-retained, multi-unit restorations on conical abutments

Cement-retained restorations

A provisional preformed plastic post, which is smooth and tapered, with an engaging hex can be shaped and screwed directly into the implant (Fig 5-7). The screw access hole is filled with temporary filling material. A conventional provisional crown can then be constructed using a matrix or polycarbonate crown form, relined with resin. The crown may then be cemented using a temporary cement. Great care should be taken to remove all excess material from the crown margin as this may lead to gingival irritation, poor healing, and a reduced aesthetic outcome. Removing the provisional restoration may be difficult at subsequent appointments, leading to fracture and the need to remake the restoration. This technique may also be used to fabricate a multi-unit provisional restoration (Fig 5-8).

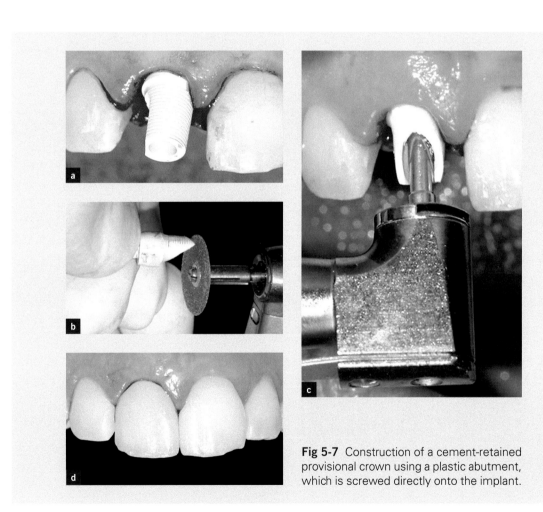

Fig 5-7 Construction of a cement-retained provisional crown using a plastic abutment, which is screwed directly onto the implant.

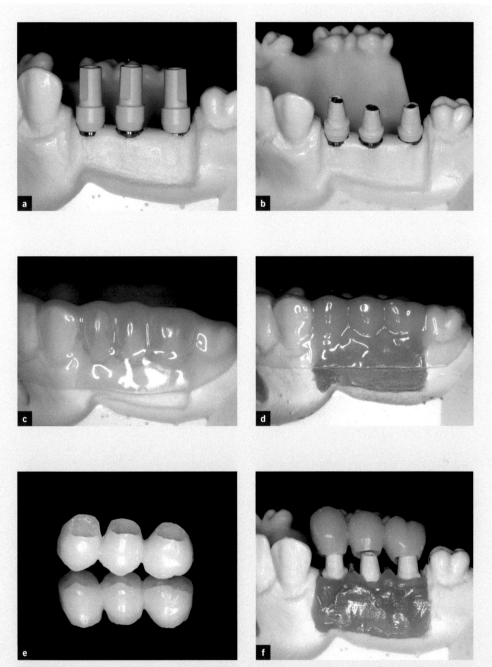

Fig 5-8 Construction of cement-retained multiple provisional restorations. A vacuum-formed matrix, based on a diagnostic waxup, is used with a self-curing resin to form the restorations on the abutments. (Courtesy of Dr. P-O Ostman)

Screw-retained restorations

A screw-retained provisional restoration may be constructed, either directly at the chairside or in the laboratory (Fig 5-9). The temporary cylinder may be metal or plastic and has grooves on its surface to allow for retention of the resin crown material. The cylinder is screwed onto the implant by means of a long waxing pin, which maintains access for the retaining screw. A hole is carefully made in the provisional crown, or crown form, so that it can be seated fully over the cylinder and waxing pin. The crown is then relined with resin, which is allowed to set *in situ*. The assembly is unscrewed from the implant, trimmed, and polished. The finished restoration is screwed directly onto the implant and the access hole filled with a pledget of cotton wool and temporary filling material. The advantage of this technique is the ease with which the provisional restoration may be removed and replaced during healing and impression taking. In addition, it is easier to modify the shape of a screw-retained provisional restoration to achieve good tissue support and healing. Since a temporary cement is not used with this technique, there are fewer problems with soft tissue irritation and inflammation.

The above types of provisional restoration are used mainly for single implant units. For multiple implant units, a non-hexed temporary cylinder should be chosen (Fig 5-10).

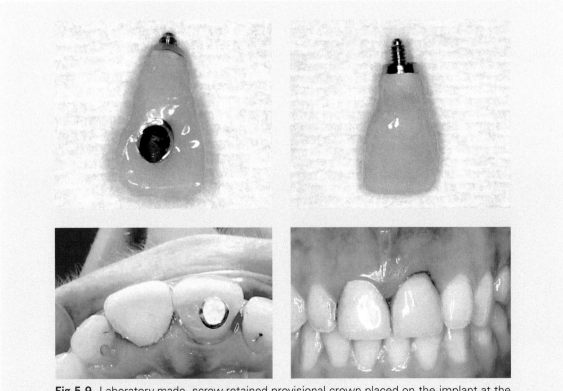

Fig 5-9 Laboratory-made, screw-retained provisional crown placed on the implant at the upper-left central incisor site.

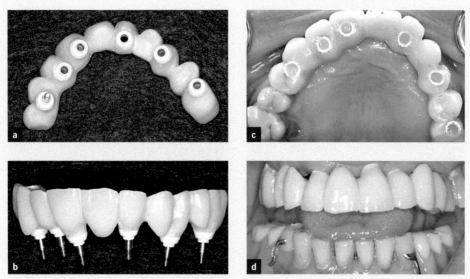

Fig 5-10 Construction of a provisional screw-retained multiple-unit restoration.

Cement-retained, multi-unit restorations on conical abutments

Conical abutments may be placed on implants to construct a multi-unit restoration. A tapered titanium coping is screwed onto the conical abutment (Fig 5-11). The coping is ridged for the retention of a plastic cap that snaps onto the coping. A vacuum-formed fixed dental prosthesis template is made in the laboratory from a diagnostic waxup. This template is filled with resin, seated over the plastic caps, and allowed to set. This step may be performed in the laboratory or directly in the mouth. Once set, the template is removed, picking up the plastic caps. The fixed dental prosthesis may then be trimmed and polished and the occlusion adjusted. The restoration is placed with temporary cement. Typically, the definitive prosthesis will be screw-retained using the conical abutments that are already in place.

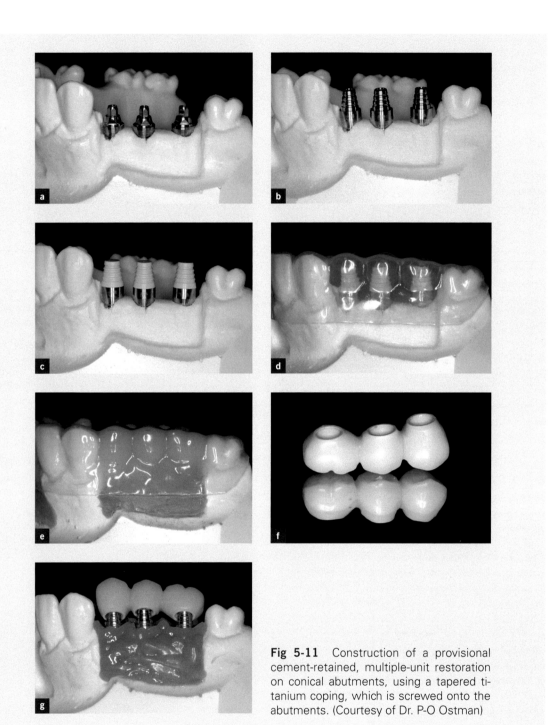

Fig 5-11 Construction of a provisional cement-retained, multiple-unit restoration on conical abutments, using a tapered titanium coping, which is screwed onto the abutments. (Courtesy of Dr. P-O Ostman)

Comparison of cement and screws as retainers for prostheses

Both cement-retained and screw-retained prostheses have been validated in clinical studies, and each type of retention has particular advantages and disadvantages (Table 5-1). Historically, screw-retained prostheses were widely used on dental implants because the restorations could be retrieved for evaluation of the underlying implants and repair of any possible complications. Cemented restorations are now widely used as they allow a more aesthetic restoration to be created. While they are not as readily retrieved as a screw-retained prosthesis, cementing restorations with provisional cement allows a degree of retrievability. There is some evidence that cement-retained fixed prostheses have fewer prosthodontic complications after delivery.

It is generally simpler to correct a misaligned implant with a cemented restoration. In the case of screw-retained restorations, if the implant is misaligned, the screw access hole may be in a variety of locations (Fig 5-12). A misaligned access hole may perforate the labial surface of the restoration or create an abnormally shaped cingulum area (Fig 5-13). This may lead to aesthetic or phonetic problems. Similarly, on a posterior tooth, the access hole may obliterate much of the occlusal anatomy (Fig 5-13). With a screw-retained prosthesis, once the retaining screw has been tightened, the access hole is filled with a resin material. During function, this material wears and stains, and periodically needs replacement. The screw access hole may represent 50% or more of the occlusal surface of a posterior tooth, so the correct occlusal contacts must be built into the resin restoration chairside.

Table 5-1 Features of cemented and screw-retained restorations.

	Cement-retained	Screw-retained
Retrievable	not easily	yes
Aesthetics	excellent	variable
Correction of misaligned implant	usually	sometimes
Ease of insertion	conventional techniques	difficult in posterior areas
Retention at minimal occlusal height	marginal	excellent
Passive fit	yes	questionable
Maintenance	minimal	moderate

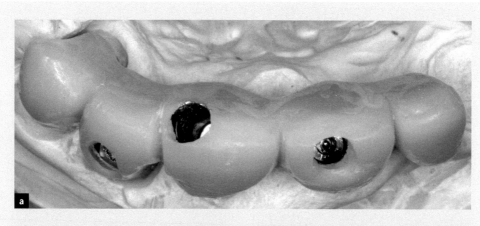

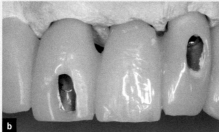
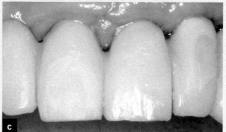

Fig 5-12 Screw access holes on an anterior implant-supported fixed dental prostheses. Alignment of implants may cause screw access to be placed buccally or a near incisal edges. Access holes may be filled with tooth-colored resin in the provisional restoration but would indicate a cemented final prothesis.

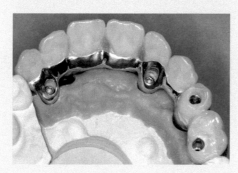

Fig 5-13 Implant placement resulting in abnormal cingulum shape and demonstrating screw access holes on the posterior teeth, which will have to be filled with resin material.

Whereas cement-retained prostheses are constructed using conventional prosthodontic procedures, screw retention requires extreme care because of the small retaining screw, which may be lost in or outside the mouth. Drivers used to tighten the retaining screws may be difficult to align in the posterior areas of the mouth. These retaining screws are also liable to loosen, being smaller than the abutment-to-implant screws and typically placed with lower torque (10 Ncm vs. 32 Ncm).

A minimum of 7 mm of space, from implant head to opposing tooth, is recommended for adequate retention of a cement-retained restoration. A screw-retained prosthesis may be provided with 4 mm of interocclusal space. Excess cement can be difficult to clear from the subgingival margin of a restoration; this can lead to persistent inflammation of the tissue. It is important that cemented restorations are designed with the prosthesis–abutment interface no more than 2–3 mm subgingival, so that excess cement may be readily removed.

Occlusal schemes for implant restorations

There is little direct evidence to suggest which type of occlusion is best for implant restorations. Where single-tooth restorations or fixed dental prostheses are provided in a partially dentate arch, it seems sensible to distribute occlusal forces between the implant restorations and natural teeth. Exactly how much force is appropriate for each depends on the number and prognosis of the remaining teeth and the length and position of the implants. In addition, unlike teeth, implants will not move in response to physiological levels of occlusal force. One popular approach to this is to ensure that the implant restorations lightly, but incompletely, hold shimstock (8–10 μm) when the teeth are just in maximum intercuspation. As the patient occludes with full force, the teeth move physiologically and the implant restorations come into heavier contact holding the shimstock along with the teeth.

It also seems reasonable to consider the amount of horizontal force transmitted to the implants via the restorations placed into function. The length of the implant, bone quality, crown–implant ratio, and evidence of parafunction are essential factors in designing the occlusal scheme. If one or more of these factors is likely to compromise the implant, it would be prudent to reduce the horizontal forces on the restoration and distribute the forces onto other implants or teeth. For example, where a long implant (>13 mm) is replacing a maxillary central incisor, with a favorable crown–implant ratio (<1), and there is no evidence of parafunction, it is acceptable to allow normal anterior guidance on this restoration. However, a shorter implant replacing a maxillary canine in a patient with bruxism would be an indication for a group function occlusion.

More extensive implant restorations generally involve fixed prostheses where the implants are rigidly splinted together, so one would expect occlusal forces to be distributed evenly among the implants. Traditionally, restorations such as the full-arch, fixed hybrid prosthesis have had very high success rates. However, where implants are placed only in the anterior part of the jaws, very high forces can be generated by posterior cantilevers on the restorations. In these situations it has been suggested that the cantilever length should be no greater than the antero-posterior spread of the supporting implants. This is typically in the order of 12–15 mm.

Selection of abutments

Abutments are components that attach directly to the head of the implant and extend through the gingiva into the oral cavity. For fixed prostheses, the abutment substitutes for the missing coronal tooth structure. A variety of abutments is available, which allows the restorative dentist to provide the patient with a restoration that is both functional and aesthetic. Some abutments are designed to be prepared directly in the mouth (or milled in the laboratory), similar to conventional crown preparations. Other abutments are customized in the laboratory and cast to their final shape. With both of these techniques the final restoration is cemented onto the finished abutment. In other designs, factory-prefabricated abutments are used and the prosthesis is screwed directly onto the abutment.

Abutment selection depends on many clinical factors and it is often not possible to make this selection until after second-stage surgery maturation of the soft tissues has occurred. In difficult situations, it is best to wait until the working cast has been made and mounted on an articulator before choosing the abutment. The abutment must take account of the position and angulation of the implant, the height and thickness of the surrounding soft tissue, the interocclusal space, and the type of restoration to be placed. Additional considerations include the height of the lip line, the occlusal scheme, and the position of the tooth in the arch.

Abutment types

The UCLA abutment

The UCLA abutment is a very versatile abutment; it may be used to produce a customized abutment for a cemented restoration, or as a screw-retained restoration.

The abutment consists of a machined gold cylinder with a plastic sleeve, which can be shaped to allow the construction of a "custom" abutment (Fig 5-14). The abutment sleeve is then waxed up in the laboratory to the shape of a core, which fits the particular tooth it is replacing, and can also be shaped to compensate for any misalignment of the implant. This design of the abutment allows for a wide range of tooth sizes and angulations to be accommodated, but with a machined fitting surface to ensure accurate fit of the abutment on the implant. The restoration may be completed on the abutment using conventional techniques (Fig 5-15).

The UCLA abutment may correct problems of implant angulation by up to 30°. This feature helps provide an aesthetic restoration by creating a substructure with a good emergence profile and contours that accurately follow the gingival tissue. The finished abutment is screwed down directly onto the implant, and a coronal restoration cemented onto the post. The UCLA abutment gives the dental technician the scope to produce an optimum abutment in the laboratory and save clinical time, particularly in challenging cases.

The UCLA abutment comes in two designs, with either a hexagonal or non-hexagonal fitting surface to engage the head of the implant. The hexagonal UCLA abutment makes for a non-rotational design that allows it to be used for single-unit restorations (Fig 5-16a). The non-hexagonal version does not engage the hexagonal top of the implant and can therefore be used for multiple-unit restorations (Fig 5-16b).

The machined collar on the UCLA abutment is 1 mm high, and so may be used where there is minimal soft tissue height above the implant head. However, in an aesthetic area, if there is a risk of metal showing through thin gingival tissue, an alternative abutment type may be preferred. Many clinicians cement fixed-implant prostheses with a temporary luting cement so that the restoration may be removed at a later date. This is useful if, for example, the abutment screw were to break or loosen. In such a case, a new screw could be placed without having to remake the prosthesis. Nonetheless, there is still a risk of damaging the prosthesis during removal, and clinical data are needed to evaluate the various approaches to implant prosthesis, design, and maintenance.

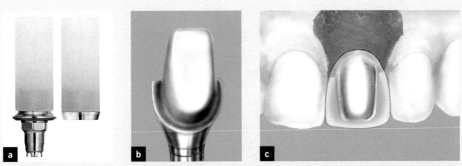

Fig 5-14 The UCLA abutment consists of a machined gold cylinder to fit the internal or external connection implant head (a).The gold cylinder is covered with a plastic sleeve, whitch may be modified by the addition of wax. The abutment is cast to create the custom abutment (b). A crown may then be constructed on the custom abutment using conventional laboratory techniques (c).

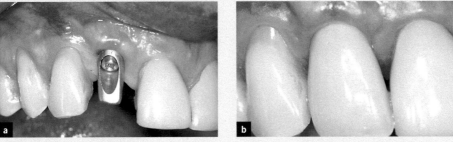

Fig 5-15 The UCLA aburment. (a) A cast custom UCLA abutment on a dental implant (b), the completed restoration is cemented onto the abutment.

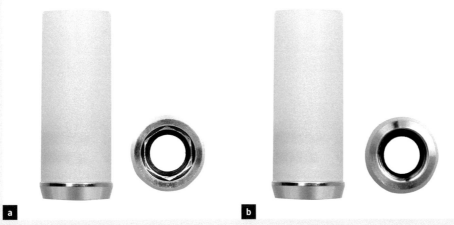

Fig 5-16 The UCLA abutments: hexed fitting surface for single-unit restorations (a) and a non-hexed fitting surface for use with mutiple-unit restorations (b). These components are for use on external hex implants.

Despite the flexibility of the UCLA abutment, the overall cost of the restoration can be high. This is because the abutment must be purchased and there is a laboratory charge for waxing and casting the abutment. The final restoration must then be fabricated on the finished abutment.

The UCLA abutment may also be used to make a screw-retained prosthesis. In this case, the abutment is waxed up to the full contour of the final restoration; this may be cut back for porcelain, if required. Hence, the abutment and restoration are one piece, and it is retained by the abutment screw (Fig 5-17). With this type of restoration, the positioning of the implant is critical, since the screw access hole should pass through the cingulum area of an anterior tooth, or the central fossa of a posterior tooth. Poor placement of the implant may lead to abnormally shaped cingulum areas or access holes that affect the occlusal morphology of posterior teeth leading to a poor occlusal relationship.

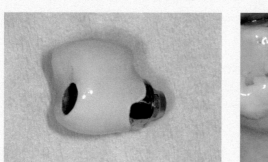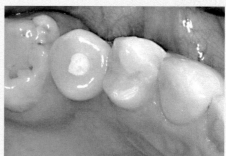

Fig 5-17 Screw-retained restoration consisting of UCLA abutment with integrated crown.

Preparable abutments

A range of implant abutments is available that can be prepared with cutting burs to the desired shape (Fig 5-18). A cement-retained prosthesis may then be made over the prepared abutments. Preparable abutments may be used for single crowns or multiple-unit restorations.

Preparable abutments are most effective where the implant placement is favorable and so there is minimal preparation to be completed on the abutment. Preparation of the abutment may be completed intraorally by the dentist or in the laboratory by the technician. Direct preparation of the abutment in the mouth is completed using the same principles as tooth preparation. Inadequate removal of post material will lead to a compromise of the final aesthetic result. It is useful to construct a silicone matrix of the fully contoured waxup as a guide to abutment preparation. This can be used in

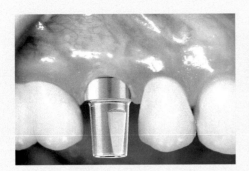
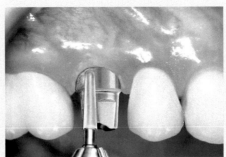
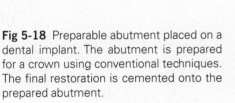
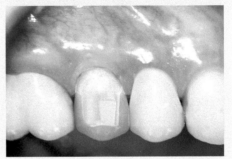

Fig 5-18 Preparable abutment placed on a dental implant. The abutment is prepared for a crown using conventional techniques. The final restoration is cemented onto the prepared abutment.

the mouth to ensure adequate reduction of the abutment for the final restoration. Similar to conventional dentistry, the abutment finish line is determined by function and aesthetics.

In order to minimize soft tissue irritation, the preparation should be finished at, or just above, the gingival margin. Where aesthetics are important, the finish line of the preparation may be 0.5–1.0 mm subgingival. The finish line for the restoration should follow the natural contours of the gingival tissue. Preparable abutments are available with different collar heights to suit the thickness of soft tissue present above the implant. The abutments may be made of metal (usually pure titanium) or of ceramic material. The latter are useful in aesthetically critical areas.

Titanium abutments

Titanium abutments may be covered with a gold-colored titanium nitride coating (Fig 5-19), which improves aesthetics, the gold color being less likely than a titanium-colored abutment to cast a grey shadow at the gingival margin. The abutment is normally machined with a 6° taper and has a pre-chamfered margin. It is available straight (Fig 5-19) or pre-angled to correct for misalignment of the implant (Fig 5-20). The abutment has a flat side to prevent rotation of the final restoration.

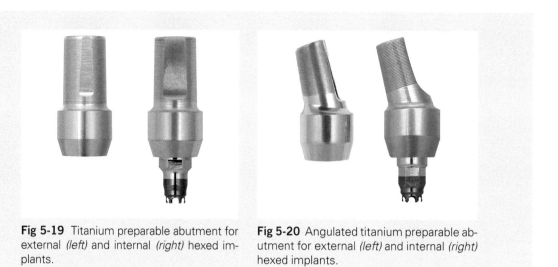

Fig 5-19 Titanium preparable abutment for external *(left)* and internal *(right)* hexed implants.

Fig 5-20 Angulated titanium preparable abutment for external *(left)* and internal *(right)* hexed implants.

Ceramic abutments

Ceramic abutments may be made of zirconia or alumina. The ceramic allows for the reflection of light in a similar way to natural teeth, and leads to less darkening of thin gingival tissue than is the case with metal. The ceramic abutment may also be preferred if a translucent material is used for the definitive prosthesis. The zirconia abutment has a machined titanium interface that fits onto the implant (Fig 5-21). The margins of the abutment can be prepared to follow the uneven contours of the gingival tissue. However, the hardness of the material can make these abutments difficult to prepare intraorally. In addition, the implant position should be close to ideal, as the abutment cannot accommodate large changes in angulation.

Prefabricated conical abutments: Screw-retained prosthesis

The conical abutment is one of several pre-machined abutments that are used for screw-retained restorations. It has a side wall taper of 15 degrees with hexagonal sides to resist rotation of the restoration, where needed (Fig 5-22). Other tapered abutments are angulated from 25 to 35 degrees to correct for the difference in orientation between implant and restoration (Fig 5-23). While the use of misaligned implants is sometimes unavoidable, it should be minimized because non-axial forces on implants and abutments are more likely to cause complications and failures.

Prefabricated abutments are manufactured with a range of collar heights to accommodate the subgingival position of the implant (Fig 5-24). Selection of the collar height will allow the margin of the restoration to be placed just below the gingival margin in order to improve the emergence profile of the final restoration. However, the abutment collar is uniform in height and does not follow the natural contours of the tissue. The screw-retained prosthesis requires a minimum of 4 mm of

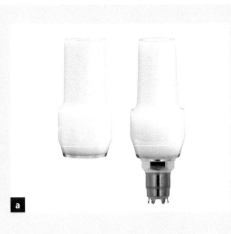

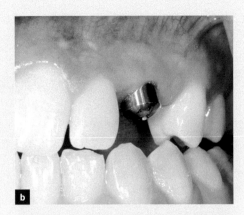

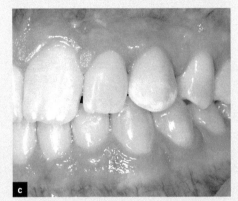

Fig 5-21 Zirconia ceramic abutments for external *(left)* and internal *(right)* hexed implants (a). Restoration of implant canine site using a ceramic abutment to minimize metal showing through the tissue (b and c).

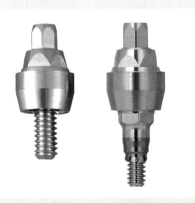

Fig 5-22 Prefabricated conical abutments for external *(left)* and internal *(right)* hexed implants.

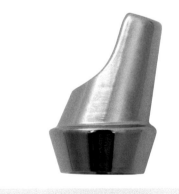

Fig 5-23 Angulated conical abutment.

103

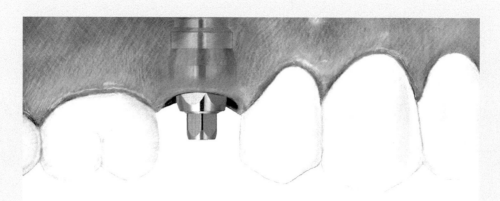

Fig 5-24 Conical abutment on dental implant showing the collar below the gingival margin.

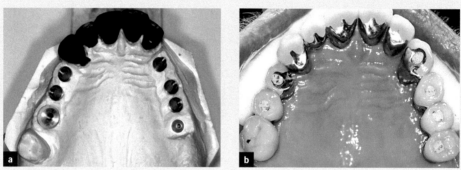

Fig 5-25 Screw-retained restorations on multiple conical abutments.

interocclusal space from the implant to the occlusal or incisal edge of the final restoration. More interocclusal space is required for the angulated abutments.

A single- or multi-unit restoration may be waxed onto a machined gold cylinder that will form the fitting surface of the prosthesis. The machined cylinder will fit the abutment more accurately than a full casting, but in either case the final prosthesis is secured with small retaining screws (Fig 5-25). The prosthesis retaining screws are much smaller than the abutment screws and are tightened to a lower torque value. The increased complexity and relative weakness of the screw-retained prosthesis mean that this type of restoration must be carefully planned, executed, and maintained.

Cement-retained prostheses

Different machined abutments are available for use with cemented prostheses. These abutments are designed for minimal modification and so can only be used when implant placement is ideal and there is ample space for the prosthesis. A parallel-sided hexagonal abutment can be used for single restorations—the crown can be fabricated directly onto a gold or ceramic coping that is machined to fit onto the abutment. The tapered abutments are generally used for multi-unit prostheses and may be straight

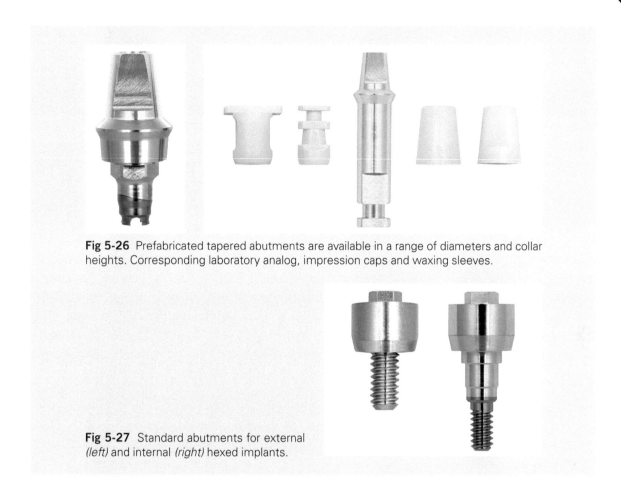

Fig 5-26 Prefabricated tapered abutments are available in a range of diameters and collar heights. Corresponding laboratory analog, impression caps and waxing sleeves.

Fig 5-27 Standard abutments for external *(left)* and internal *(right)* hexed implants.

or angulated (Fig 5-26). Despite the simplicity and cost-effectiveness of using stock components, these prefabricated abutments have not commonly been used due to their lack of flexibility.

The standard abutment

The original abutment for the external hexagon implant was the standard abutment. This two-piece abutment consists simply of a cylinder and a screw, and its purpose was to provide a restorative platform above the soft tissue level (Fig 5-27). The standard abutment requires a minimum of 2 mm tissue height and is available up to 7 mm high. Standard abutments now have few indications, though they may be used for the fabrication of full-arch, fixed hybrid prostheses. For this purpose, a secondary cylinder, which is screwed onto the standard abutment, is incorporated into the prosthesis framework. The standard abutment may also act as the platform for some overdenture attachments.

One disadvantage of the standard abutment is that the collar has a uniform height and so does not follow the natural contours of the gingival margin. This feature makes it difficult to achieve an appropriate emergence profile and acceptable aesthetics. As with other intermediate-type abutments, it also necessitates the cost and complexity of a second restorative component and screw.

Custom-machined abutments

Advances in computer-assisted design, computer-assisted manufacture (CAD/CAM) have made it possible to manufacture precision custom abutments (Fig 5-28). Based on an impression of the implant, the CAD/CAM system allows for the design of individual abutments by computer, or the scanning of an abutment waxup. The specifications for the abutment are then transmitted to a central factory, where a metal or ceramic abutment is machined, and then returned to the local laboratory. The advantage of this approach is that the abutment can take into account implant angulation, tissue height, and the size and contour of the final restoration (Fig 5-28). Because it is a one-step process, the custom machined abutment eliminates the need to buy a stock abutment and then modify it in the laboratory. The centralization of the manufacturing process means that the abutments can be produced with an accurate fit.

A further option is available to construct a final custom abutment based on the use of a special two-piece healing abutment. This healing abutment has codes embedded on its occlusal surface containing the information necessary to create the final abutment (Fig 5-29). It provides the position of the implant hex, the soft tissue height, and the implant platform diameter. A simple conventional elastomeric impression is made of the healing abutment, ensuring reproduction of the coded area. The master cast is scanned in a CAD/CAM laboratory where an abutment is designed and milled. A crown may then be constructed and returned to the dentist for insertion. This system eliminates the need for implant-level impressions and simplifies the restorative technique.

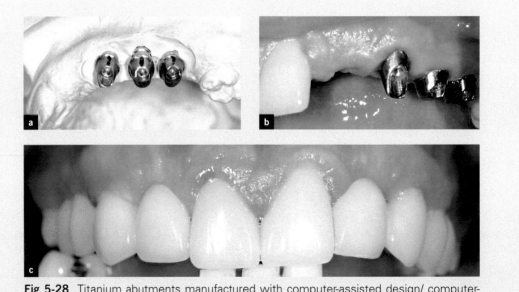

Fig 5-28 Titanium abutments manufactured with computer-assisted design/ computer-assisted technology. The abutments on a cast (a) and placed on the dental implants (b). Final restoration cemented in place (c).

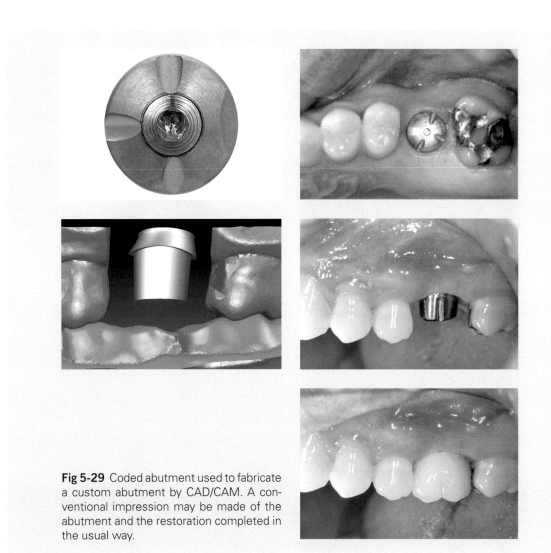

Fig 5-29 Coded abutment used to fabricate a custom abutment by CAD/CAM. A conventional impression may be made of the abutment and the restoration completed in the usual way.

Instruments and Components

It is essential that the restorative dentist has a complete understanding of the components that are going to be utilized in any implant restorative treatment. This will allow a successful, functional, and aesthetic restoration to be constructed in a predictable manner.

Drivers

Drivers and placement instruments are used for abutments and other restorative components to be placed on osseointegrated implants. All the drivers are designed to carry different types of components to the mouth for easier placement and removal. Most are available in short versions for use in the posterior parts of the mouth where space is limited. Longer versions are available for use anteriorly and where the crown length necessitates a longer driver.

Hexagonal-headed driver (hex driver)

The main uses for this type of driver are removal and placement of titanium healing abutments, the tightening and loosening of the guide pins in the pick-up type of impression copings, and the tightening and loosening of hexagonal-headed abutment screws (Fig 6-1).

Square-headed driver

The square-headed driver is used mainly for tightening the square-headed abutment screws (Fig 6-2). These screws have the advantage that they can be used with greater torque than the hexagonal screws.

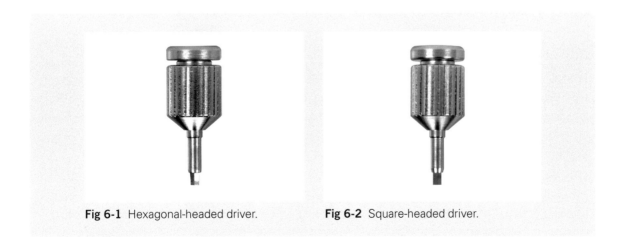

Fig 6-1 Hexagonal-headed driver.   **Fig 6-2** Square-headed driver.

Abutment driver

The abutment driver is used to tighten the central screw of a conical abutment while the collar is being held on to the hexagon of the implant by the conical abutment placement instrument (Fig 6-3).

Contra-angle torque driver

This is a contra-angle, manually operated driver with interchangeable torque controllers (Fig 6-4). This driver is able to apply the appropriate torque for the screw. The main advantage of this torque driver is that it can be used in reverse to remove screws that have been tightened.

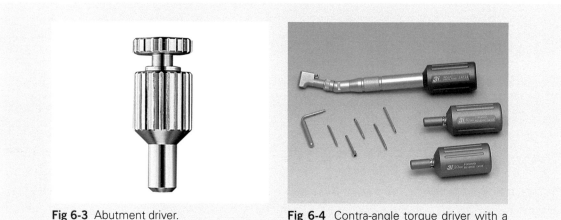

Fig 6-3 Abutment driver.

Fig 6-4 Contra-angle torque driver with a selection of tips and torque controllers.

Restorative torque drivers

The amount of torque that is placed on a screw is critical to the stability of any abutment-implant assembly. This leads to long-term success of the restoration. A restorative torque driver allows the clinician to place the necessary amount of torque when the screw is tightened (Fig 6-5). It consists of a handle and a circular head that can accept all contra-angle latch grip tips. On the underside there is an outer border that is marked with a triangle and a diamond. The inner surface has three triangles marked. As the torque driver is rotated and the inner and outer triangles align, 20 Ncm of torque are applied to the screw. As the driver is further rotated, the inner triangles and the outer diamonds become coincident and 35 Ncm are applied. The torque driver is accurate to 2 Ncm and is easy to use. It is important to note that hand tightening alone is not sufficient to provide the correct amount of preload required to give total stability to the abutment-implant assembly. Screw loosening will be far more common where arbitrary hand tightening is used.

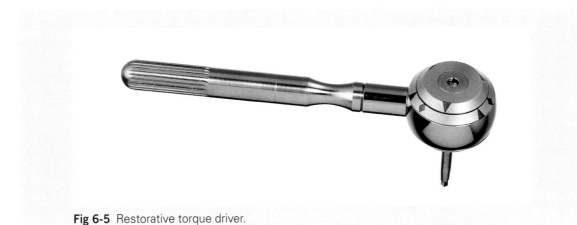

Fig 6-5 Restorative torque driver.

Provisional healing abutments

Provisional healing abutments are made in varying heights and diameters to be used in multiple situations (Fig 6-6). Some healing abutments are flared and matched to the mesiodistal diameter of natural teeth at the tissue level. This allows the gingival tissue to heal around the abutment and gives the final restoration the correct emergence profile as it exits out of the gingival to create an aesthetic restoration. The healing abutment also allows the full visualization of the implant seating surface, which makes impression taking easier and allows all the components to engage the implant surface for a more reliable and precise fit.

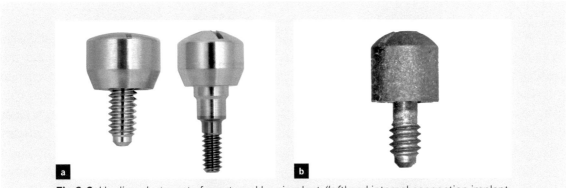

Fig 6-6 Healing abutments for external hex implant *(left)* and internal connection implant *(right)* may be flared to achieve a smooth emergence profile from implant to crown (a). Parallel-sided healing abutments are also available for the replacement of narrow diameter teeth (b).

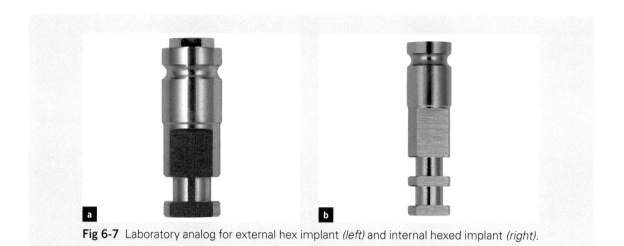

Fig 6-7 Laboratory analog for external hex implant *(left)* and internal hexed implant *(right)*.

Laboratory analogs

These are metal replicas that duplicate the implant head or abutment connected to the implant (Fig 6-7). They are used in the laboratory to construct a working model.

Impression copings

Impression copings have been designed for final impression taking after the soft tissue has matured (Fig 6-8). These impression copings have the same flare as the healing abutments and fully support the soft tissue around the head of the implant. The most commonly used impression copings are the "pick-up" type, which are screwed down onto the head of the implant and secured by means of an internal guide pin. The impression is then made in a tray where a hole had been made to allow access to the guide pin. Once the material has set, the guide pin is disengaged, leaving the coping embedded in the impression. This is also known as the "open tray" impression technique. An implant analog is screwed onto the impression coping, and from this assembly a working model is constructed.

An alternative technique for making implant impressions is to use a "transfer-type" impression coping (Fig 6-9). The coping is screwed onto the implant and an impression is made. Once set, the impression is removed, leaving the impression coping still connected to the implant. The coping is unscrewed and connected to a laboratory analog. This assembly is then relocated into the impression so that a working model may be constructed. This is known as the "closed tray" impression technique, since no hole is made in the impression tray. The disadvantage of this technique is the difficulty of accurately repositioning the copings in the impression.

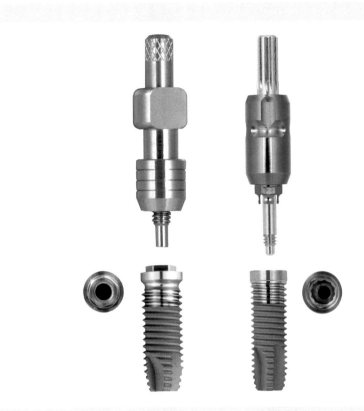

Fig 6-8 Pick-up impression copings for external hex implant *(left)* and internal hexed implant *(right)*.

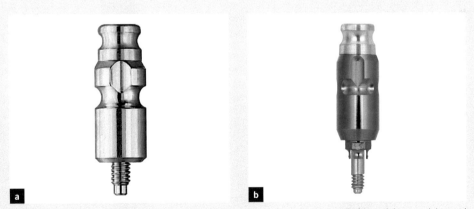

Fig 6-9 Transfer impression copings for external hex implant *(left)* and internal hexed implant *(right)*.

Screws

Abutment screw and preload

This is used to clamp the abutment of choice to the implant and create a rigid assembly (Fig 6-10). A predetermined torque is applied to the screw, which is intended to stretch the screw to 80% of its elastic limit. This stretching of the screw (preload) creates compressive forces within the implant screw assembly and hence creates a clamping together of the abutment and the implant at the interface. To improve the clamping force achieved, some manufacturers coat screws with dry lubricants, such as 24-carat gold or carbon. Abutment screws are manufactured either with a hexagonal or square head to facilitate ease of transmission of the correct preload through the screw. These screws should be torqued as per the manufacturer's instructions. It is recommended that a higher torque (35 Ncm) be applied to the abutment screws on external hex implants. This is to ensure a stable connection between the abutment and implant.

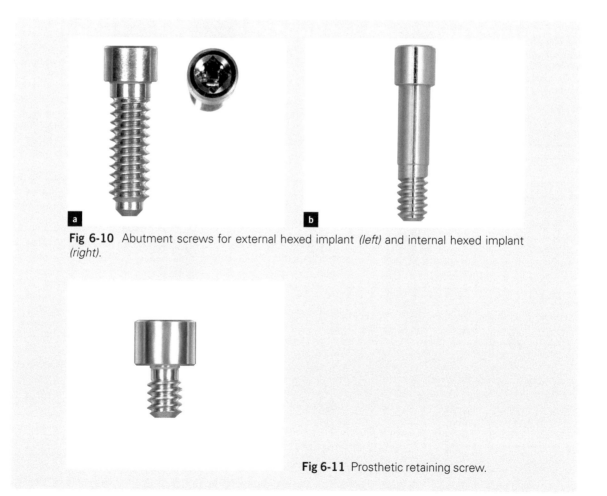

Fig 6-10 Abutment screws for external hexed implant *(left)* and internal hexed implant *(right)*.

Fig 6-11 Prosthetic retaining screw.

Retaining screw

The retaining screw is used to clamp the final prosthesis to an intermediate abutment, such as a conical or standard abutment. These screws are typically smaller than abutment screws and are placed with less torque (Fig 6-11). They should be torqued as per the manufacturer's instructions.

Temporary cylinders

Temporary cylinders are used to fabricate provisional prostheses. They are available in metal or plastic versions, for internal and external hex implants (Fig 6-12).

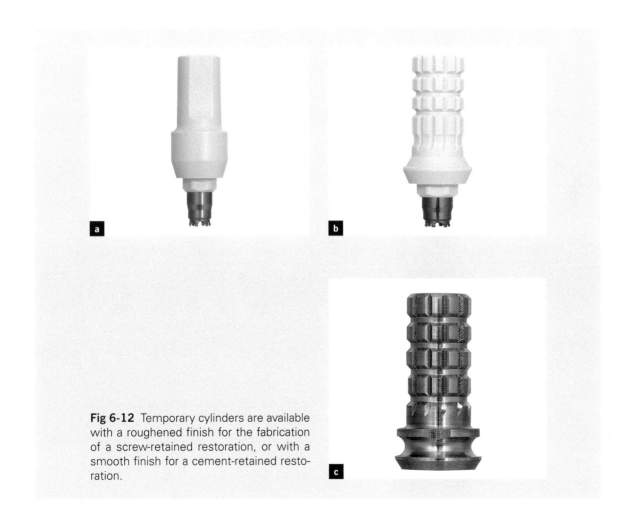

Fig 6-12 Temporary cylinders are available with a roughened finish for the fabrication of a screw-retained restoration, or with a smooth finish for a cement-retained restoration.

CHAPTER
7

Overdentures

Conventional complete dentures do not satisfy many patients because of limitations in function and comfort. While edentulism is decreasing in western populations, patients are living longer and are more subject to alveolar bone resorption. Hence, the number of edentulous people in the population may not be decreasing. At the same time, many elderly patients may have reduced ability to wear dentures as a result of illness or medications. For these reasons, implant-supported overdentures have become an attractive alternative to conventional dentures, particularly in the mandible. The purpose of implants is to stabilize the overdenture: the prosthesis will still move during function if it is partly tissue borne. Hence it is essential that the overdenture is made according to best practice for complete denture construction. The addition of dental implants will not compensate for a poorly fitting denture.

Recent studies have indicated that the provision of comfortable and functional complete dentures improves the quality of life of patients. Often successful denture therapy can only be achieved by the addition of dental implants to provide retention and stability for the denture. The main disadvantages of implant overdentures are the surgical procedure involved and the need for ongoing maintenance of the implants and attachments.

The indications for overdentures are:
- patients having edentulous jaws, especially with opposing natural teeth, where removable dentures are unstable
- patients having difficulty wearing complete or partial dentures
- remaining teeth having a poor prognosis
- atrophic alveolus with inadequate supporting tissues
- patients having poor neuromuscular control
- patients needing additional confidence (actors, singers)
- mental foramina at, or close to, the crest of the residual alveolar ridge
- strong mentalis muscle activity
- retruded tongue position
- decreased salivary flow.

The contraindications for overdentures are:
- inability to undergo implant surgery
- psychiatric disorders
- inability to consent to treatment
- insufficient alveolar bone (minimum of 8 mm needed)
- local infection, roots, or other disease at the implant site
- generalized bone disease
- patient wanting a fixed restoration
- inability to maintain hygiene around the implants.

Mandibular overdenture

A minimum of one implant is required on each side of the mandible, anterior to the mental foramina. The overdenture may attach to each implant individually, or the two implants may be joined by a bar. Clips or attachments in the denture then retain it to the implants. The use of implants with individual attachments is simpler, less expensive, and as effective as the use of a bar-retained overdenture. With an implant-stabilized overdenture, patients can usually expect improvements in chewing, comfort, and confidence. However, they should be advised that the prosthesis will not be "like their own teeth." Patients who have recently become edentulous, and have never successfully worn a removable denture, are more likely to expect a prosthesis that does not move at all. In contrast, those who have worn dentures but have gradually lost supporting tissues are likely to appreciate the increased stability and comfort of an overdenture. Studies have demonstrated that this mode of treatment may significantly improve the quality of life for many edentulous patients.

Assessment of patients for overdentures

Many of the same principles apply to the placement of implants for overdentures as for fixed restorations. A thorough history and clinical examination are completed, and radiographs are taken. The restorative clinician should pay particular attention to the arch form and the shape of the residual alveolar ridge. A panoramic radiograph and lateral cephalograph are generally sufficient to plan implant placement in the mandible. Longer implants are desirable, and implants of regular diameter are used as standard. Since most overdentures are provided for patients with moderate to severe alveolar resorption, there is usually sufficient vertical space for the implant abutment and overdenture attachment.

Care must be taken with the buccolingual position of implants. The implants should ideally be placed in the long axis of the denture teeth, to minimize tipping forces on the overdenture and to allow for sufficient restorative space. Because alveolar resorption occurs facially as well as vertically, the center of the residual ridge is usually lingual to the teeth. If implants are placed in this position, they may cause excessive bulk on the lingual surface of the denture and compromise denture function. Moreover, alveolar resorption often leaves the mandibular residual ridge retroclined, which can be visualized on the lateral cephalograph. This characteristic makes it difficult to place implants upright in the correct position.

Clinical procedures for overdentures

The steps involved in making an implant-retained overdenture are shown in Fig 7-1. A surgical guide for implant placement can be readily made using the patient's conventional denture. For patients without a denture, it is advisable to fabricate a denture to establish the extensions, vertical dimension and tooth position, before proceeding with implant placement. An existing denture may be used

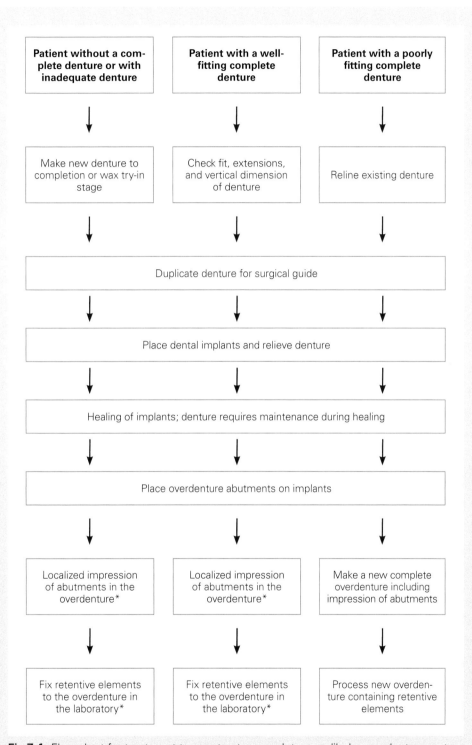

Fig 7-1 Flow chart for treatment to construct a complete mandibular overdenture on two independent implant abutments. *Alternatively, the retentive elements can be fixed to the overdenture intraorally with acrylic resin.

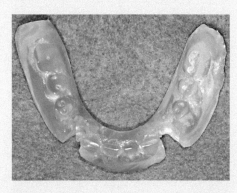

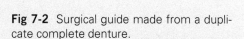
Fig 7-2 Surgical guide made from a duplicate complete denture.

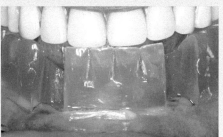
Fig 7-3 Try-in of surgical guide for a mandibular overdenture.

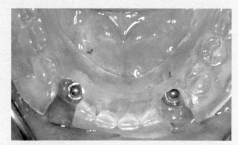
Fig 7-4 Checking the implant position using the surgical guide.

as a guide to implant placement, provided that the teeth are in the correct position and the base is properly extended.

The complete denture may readily be duplicated in clear acrylic resin to use as a surgical guide (Fig 7-2). The desired position of the implants is then marked on the guide. Since overdentures will rotate around the axis between the implants, the implants should be placed near the corners of the arch, particularly if a bar is to be used.

A notch is cut in the facial side of the guide, which will allow a hole to be drilled in the alveolar ridge as close as possible to the long axis of the denture teeth (Fig 7-2). At a minimum, the implant abutment and the denture attachment must fit within the boundaries of the denture at that site, both horizontally and vertically. It is important that the implants be placed in attached mucosa, which is usually near the crest of the residual ridge. This can be checked in the patient's mouth using the surgical guide (Fig 7-3). The guide may be used to verify the correct placement of the implants (Fig 7-4).

If it is not possible to place implants in the ideal position, then the guide can be modified further to find alternative implant sites. If an implant is placed on thin, moveable mucosa, the tissue may remain inflamed and painful. This situation may warrant a free gingival graft to the site.

Once the implant is placed, a patient should not wear the complete denture for at least a week, to allow healing to begin. When the sutures are removed, the fitting surface of the denture is relieved 2–3 mm at the surgical site and relined with a soft lining material. The patient should be seen no more than 6 weeks after surgery to check the healing of tissues and to replace the soft lining in the denture.

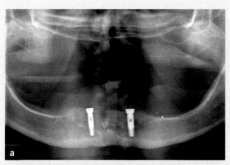
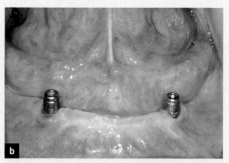

Fig 7-5 Radiograph of mandibular implants (a), and the Locator abutments in place (b). Abutments are available in different heights; they should protrude 3–4 mm above the soft tissue.

Fig 7-6 Locator attachments are placed in the denture by first relieving the fitting surface over the abutments. Retentive inserts of various strengths come in different colors and the Locator instrument is useful for changing the inserts in the housing.

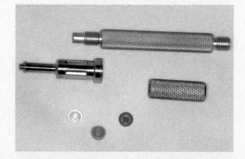

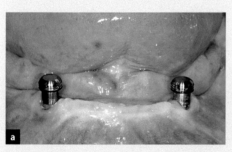
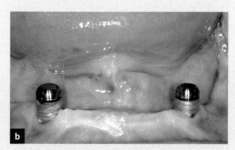

Fig 7-7 Locator attachments are placed onto the abutments in the mouth (a). To prevent the overdenture from locking in, the abutments may be blocked out using small elastic bands (b). The attachments are then picked up in the denture using cold-cure acrylic resin (c).

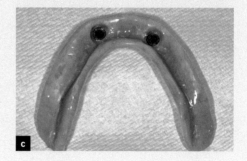

Abutments may be attached to the implants approximately 3–4 months following placement (Fig 7-5). At this point, the overdenture is then fitted with attachments to provide added stability and retention (Figs 7-6 and 7-7).

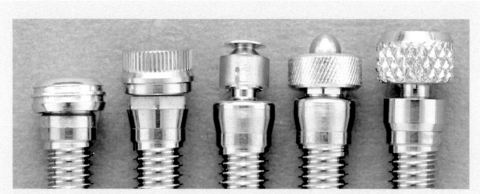

Fig 7-8 Different types of overdenture attachment that can be used with implants.

Overdenture attachments

A variety of attachments are available to connect overdentures to implants (Fig 7-8). Most of these are based on existing systems that were used for tooth-borne overdentures.

The use of an attachment should be considered in terms of:
- size of components: height and bulk of the assembly
- ease of placement of the retentive element in the overdenture base
- ability to easily adjust the retention of the assembly
- frequency of component failure
- rate of wear: loss of retention of components
- ease of replacement of retentive elements
- cost.

Studies have shown that maintenance of overdentures can be a significant drawback for patients and clinicians, so reliability of the attachments and ease of replacement are key factors.

Locator attachments

A simple and cost-effective method of providing the patient with an implant-retained overdenture is the use of Locator attachments (Figs 7-5 to 7-7). These are self-aligning and have a low vertical height, giving maximum stability. They consist of a one-piece abutment, which does not engage the implant hex. It has a triangular recess on top to which the female component fits. The retentive component is held within a metal housing, which is processed into the denture base either in the laboratory or at the chairside. The female retentive component is made of nylon and is available in different retentive strengths, which are color coded for convenience. Locator attachments may also be used with maxillary overdentures to increase retention (Fig 7-9), although, more commonly, at least four implants are placed in the maxilla to support a removable or fixed prosthesis.

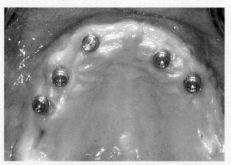 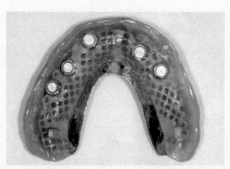

Fig 7-9 Maxillary implant-retained overdenture using five Locator abutments. Maxillary overdentures generally incorporate metal substructures to reduce bulk and increase strength.

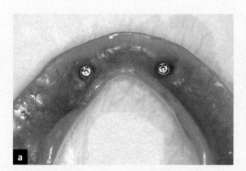 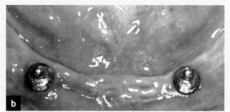

Fig 7-10 Ball abutments on the implants (a) and the female attachments in the overdenture (b).

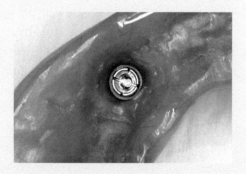

Fig 7-11 The leaves of the female attachment can be adjusted to vary the amount of retention achieved.

Ball (or stud) abutment

Another popular overdenture attachment is the ball (or stud) abutment. Both the male and female parts of the assembly are typically metal, and so they are robust and hard wearing (Fig 7-10). The leaves on the female attachment can be adjusted to increase retention (Fig 7-11), but when the component wears, the entire attachment must be replaced.

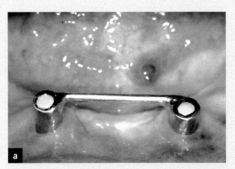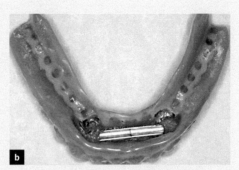

Fig 7-12 Bar-retained mandibular overdenture showing the bar in place (a) and the intaglio of the overdenture (b).

Bar-retained overdentures

A bar may be used to provide good support and retention for an overdenture instead of independent abutments. The bar is soldered onto customized (UCLA) abutments. It is important to remember that the tissue supporting the overdenture is compressible and so movement of the prosthesis will occur during function.

When two implants are placed in the mandible, a straight bar should be used in order to allow rotation of the overdenture around the bar during function (Fig 7-12). The implants must be placed in the alveolar ridge so as to allow for a straight bar between the implants that is long enough to hold a retentive clip (approximately 7 mm), but which will not interfere with the tongue.

The cross-section of the bar should allow for some rotation of the retentive clip. An oval-shaped bar, such as a Dolder bar, is useful in this respect. The retentive clips in the overdenture will wear over time and need to be adjusted. Sometimes the clips detach from the overdenture and a new clip must be added intraorally or in the laboratory. One disadvantage of the bar-retained overdenture is that the whole bar must be removed from the patient and returned to the laboratory for any further processing. When independent abutments are used with an overdenture, an impression may be made of the abutments or at implant level, and stock components used for the laboratory stages.

As an alternative to the above design with two implants, four or more implants may be placed to support a removable overdenture (Fig 7-13). In this case, rotation of the overdenture on the supporting bar does not occur and the prosthesis is essentially implant supported. The overdenture must have adequate strength to resist occlusal forces, and distal extensions used with care to avoid excessive torquing of the bar and implants.

The fabrication of a bar-retained overdenture is similar to that with independent abutments, although there is an extra step for construction of the bar itself. It is usually necessary to make a new

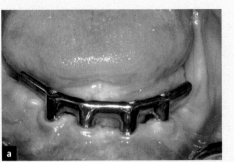

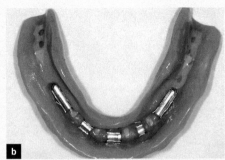

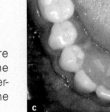

Fig 7-13 Implant-supported overdenture using a bar on four implants, showing the bar in the mouth (a), the intaglio of the over-denture with retentive clips (b), and the overdenture in place (c).

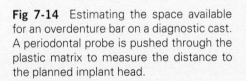

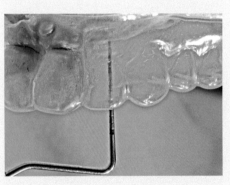

Fig 7-14 Estimating the space available for an overdenture bar on a diagnostic cast. A periodontal probe is pushed through the plastic matrix to measure the distance to the planned implant head.

denture to fit over the bar, rather than adapting an existing complete denture, because of the bulk of the bar. In the planning phase, it is important to check that there is sufficient space to accommodate the bar and its retentive elements without increasing the bulk of the denture palatally. The space available for the bar may be measured using a matrix of the diagnostic waxup placed on a cast (Fig 7-14).

The use of CAD/CAM technology allows for the construction of machined bars directly on the implants (Fig 7-15a). The bars can be made in a variety of cross-sectional designs, and primary retention is achieved using clips or a retentive sleeve (Fig 7-15b). Overdenture bars can include additional retentive elements at the request of the restorative clinician (Fig 7-16).

Construction of machined bar-supported overdentures involves the same clinical stages as outlined in Fig 7-1, although the laboratory phase is simplified as it eliminates the need for casting or soldering components. The procedure for construction of a machined bar to retain an overdenture is as in Fig 7-1 up to the healing stage. After this, the following steps are followed:

- complete denture impression including implants with Verification Index
- laboratory fabrication of bar using matrix of the existing denture or wax try-in as a guide to placement
- intraoral try-in of bar (section bar and solder or weld, if required)
- wax try-in of overdenture
- processing of overdenture containing retentive clips (alternatively, the retentive clips can be fixed to the overdenture intraorally with acrylic resin).

It is important to fully check a new implant-stabilized overdenture at time of delivery in the same way as a conventional complete denture. The base should be checked for areas of tissue impingement and the patient should be seen within a few days for follow-up. Thereafter, patients with overdentures should be seen on a regular maintenance and recall schedule to check for tissue health, function, implant integrity, and status of the retentive components.

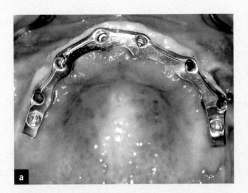
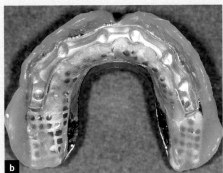

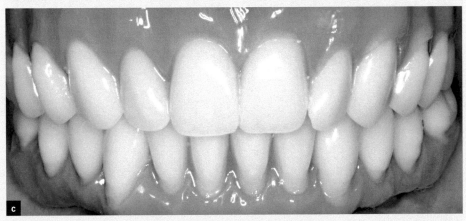

Fig 7-15 Parallel-sided machined bar to support and retain a maxillary overdenture (a). There are two sites to place retentive attachments in the bar, should they be needed. The electrolytically formed retentive sleeve in the fitting surface of the overdenture (try-in, b) fits on to the bar. (c) The finished overdenture in position.

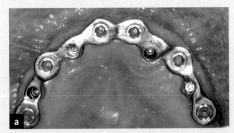
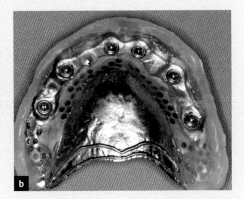

Fig 7-16 An implant-retained machined titanium bar to accomodate six Ceka attachments (a). The corresponding overdenture try-in with the attachments in place (b).

131

CHAPTER 8

Immediate Loading of Implants

The immediate loading of single or multiple dental implants is used to reduce overall treatment times and increase patients' acceptance of implant treatment. Immediate loading eliminates the use of a removable prosthesis and at no time is the patient without teeth. This provides excellent psychological benefits as the patient has a fixed prosthesis fitted at the same appointment as implant placement. It also eliminates the need for second-stage surgery. However, the technique requires longer chair-side time on the day of the procedure and good coordination between the surgeon and restorative clinician.

Apart from the standard two-stage procedure, alternative protocols have been proposed for the restoration of implants soon after their placement. These approaches have been complicated by varied use of terms such as "immediate loading" and "early loading." It could be considered that immediate loading means functional loading of a restoration within 24 hours of implant placement. This approach may be used where there is good bone quality and good primary stability of the implant(s) on placement. Available evidence indicates that immediate loading is as successful as the conventional protocol under these circumstances. It is prudent to avoid immediate loading if bone height and width are limited, or there are parafunctional habits or patient health complications.

Early loading of implants refers to restorations placed from one day to three weeks after implant surgery. There is less evidence to support the use of this technique, as bone remodeling around implants is beginning during this period. There is evidence for a "stability dip" of implants between about three weeks and six weeks after placement, as the bone surrounding the implants is resorbing and new bone is not yet formed. Hence, it is best to avoid placing restorations during this period. Early loading also seems to afford less advantage to patients when compared with immediate loading protocols and the former is used infrequently.

The concept of immediate restoration without loading is favored by some authors, although it is not certain that implants can be restored without any functional loading, even if the restorations are not in occlusion. An extension of this concept is progressive loading of implants, which suggests that the restorations are not bearing occlusal load at first; the loading is increased gradually over the following months as the surrounding bone remodels. This entails progressive additions to provisional restorations, but the technique has not been shown to be more successful than other loading protocols.

Multiple implants

Because of the quality of bone and the generally good stability of implants in the interforaminal region of the mandible, immediate loading is more often carried out in this area, with the implants splinted together. The technique can be applied at the time of tooth extraction, so the patient may go directly from having teeth to a fixed prosthesis. For a full-arch restoration, between four and six implants should be placed, and these should have the greatest anteroposterior spread that can be achieved. A more favorable result is likely in a curved arch than in a flattened arch as the former allows for better stress distribution in the restoration and the use of a distal cantilever.

Placement technique

A complete mandibular denture is made before implant placement using conventional techniques (Fig 8-1). It is helpful if the denture is thicker, buccolingually, than normal to ensure there is sufficient acrylic resin to accommodate the implant components.

Following the complete planning phase, including the necessary radiographs, implants are placed in the usual way. The denture itself, or a modified copy, may be used as a surgical guide (Fig 8-2).

Once the stability of the implants is verified, the immediate occlusal loading abutments are torqued directly onto the implants. Abutments should be selected so they are at least 1 mm above the soft tissue.

Provisional cylinders with retentive features are then screwed onto the abutments (Fig 8-3). If a distal extension of the prosthesis is required, it can be supported by a titanium arm that is fixed to the most distal provisional cylinder.

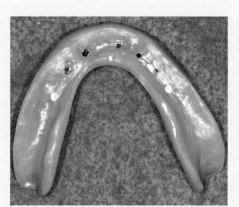

Fig 8-1 A complete denture is made with appropriate aesthetics and occlusion, but thicker buccolingually to allow for implant placement, as marked.

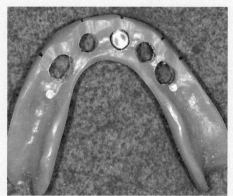

Fig 8-2 Guide holes for implant placement are made in the denture.

The provisional cylinders have a notch at their base to support a sheet of rubber dam that separates the surgical and restorative sites (Fig 8-4). The denture is modified so that it can accommodate the provisional cylinders and distal extensions. Seating of the denture is verified by checking the occlusal contacts.

Once this is done, cold-cure acrylic resin is placed around the cylinders, connecting them firmly to the denture (Fig 8-5). When the resin is set, the cylinders are unscrewed from the abutments and the prosthesis removed from the mouth. The prosthesis is then trimmed and finished, either at the chairside or in the laboratory.

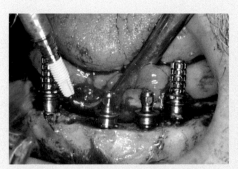

Fig 8-3 Implant insertion using the osteotomies made with the surgical guide. The two distal implants have abutments and provisional cylinders in place.

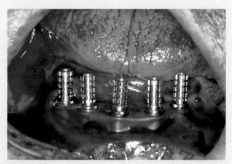

Fig 8-4 Provisional cylinders in place with rubber dam barrier.

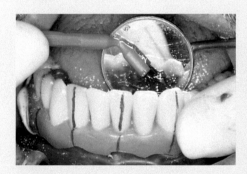

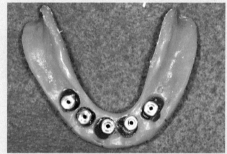

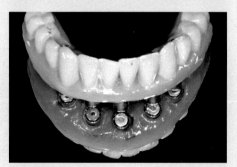

Fig 8-5 Cold-cure resin used to attach the denture to the provisional cylinders. The prosthesis is then removed and taken to the laboratory for finishing. (Courtesy of Dr. Seamus Sharkey)

The fitting surface of the prosthesis should be at least 2 mm from the soft tissue to allow for cleaning by the patient (Fig 8-6). The screw access holes are filled with cotton wool and a provisional restorative material.

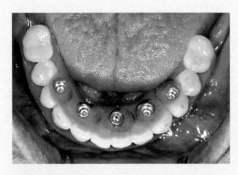

Fig 8-6 Provisional prosthesis fitted and occlusion verified. There should be space between the prosthesis and tissue for cleaning by the patient.

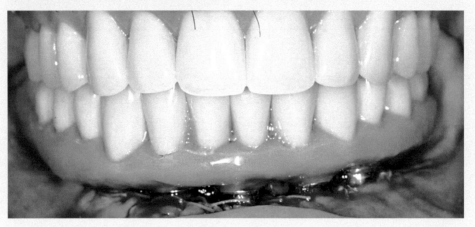

Once the provisional prosthesis is in place, the patient is instructed on cleaning and maintenance of the restoration. The prosthesis can be readily removed to check for appropriate healing (Fig 8-7). After 8–12 weeks, a definitive prosthesis can be constructed for the patient.

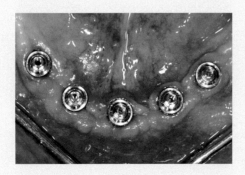

Fig 8-7 Healing of the tissues 4 weeks after implant placement.

The definitive prosthesis consists of a machined or cast metal substructure overlayed with denture teeth and acrylic resin. This prosthesis is screwed onto the abutments. This type of restoration is usually termed a 'fixed hybrid prosthesis'. Use of CAD/CAM technology simplifies the construction of the metal substructure for the definitive prosthesis. An impression is made of the implants or abutments and the master cast is verified for accuracy (Fig 8-8).

Once completed, a bar of various designs can be machined from titanium and returned for completion (Fig 8-9). This eliminates the need for complex laboratory procedures, such as casting and soldering. In addition, titanium has the advantage of being lighter and less expensive than gold alloys.

The prosthesis is carefully checked for fit, occlusion, and aesthetics. Oral hygiene procedures are checked, particularly that the patient can clean the fitting surface of the prosthesis with brushes and/or floss (Fig 8-10).

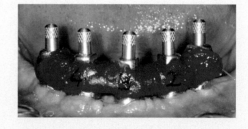

Fig 8-8 Taking an impression of the implants for the final prosthesis.

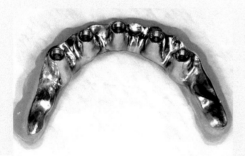

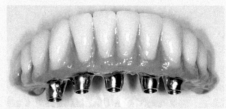

Fig 8-9 Hybrid prosthesis consisting of denture teeth processed with acrylic resin to a milled titanium framework.

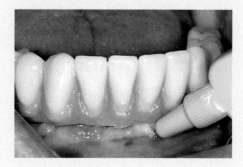

Fig 8-10 Cleaning the fitting surface of the prosthesis with an interdental brush.

Single implants

Single implants can be immediately restored provided that the implant meets the criteria outlined above. This is usually done in the aesthetic zone and may follow the immediate extraction of the tooth to be replaced. A provisional restoration is made according to the procedure described in Chapter 5. The placement of an immediate restoration facilitates the optimum healing of the soft tissue, creating an aesthetic result. As discussed above, a screw-retained crown will be more favorable than a cement-retained restoration. It is important to check that there is little or no occlusal contact on an immediate restoration in the intercuspal position and in lateral excursions. A definitive restoration may be made once tissue healing and maturation have occurred.

PART II

Practical Protocols

Note to the reader

In the following chapters concerning practical protocols in implant restoration, figures will be provided side-by-side to illustrate both internal and external connection types. Internal hex connections will be presented on the right-hand side and external on the left, as indicated at the top of each page.

CHAPTER

9

Single-tooth Restoration Using a Direct Technique with a Preparable Abutment

external		internal

Materials and components

- metal or ceramic abutment
- final abutment retaining screw
- square driver
- hexagonal driver
- gauze
- periodontal probe or measuring post
- torque indicator
- square or hex tip to go into indicator

- burs (H33L.31.021, 703L.FG and H158.31.012 H297FG)
- retraction cord
- impression material
- adhesive
- custom or stock impression
- immediate restorative material
- bite registration material

Procedure

At second-stage implant surgery, a flared healing abutment is placed on the implant and the tissues are allowed to heal. The healing abutment should be visible at least 1 mm above the level of the soft tissue (Fig 9-1).

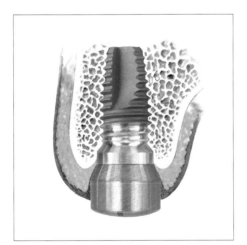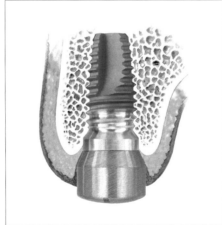

Fig 9-1 Implant after healing period at second-stage surgery with healing abutment in place.

Remove the healing abutment using a hexagonal screwdriver (Figs 9-2 and 9-3). It is useful to place a square of gauze behind the operating area as the components are quite small and it prevents possible loss of the abutment if the patient swallows.

external	internal

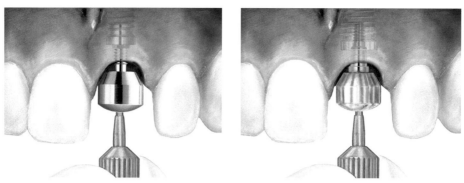

Fig 9-2 Healing abutment removed using hexagonal driver.

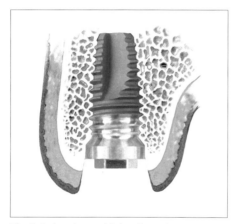 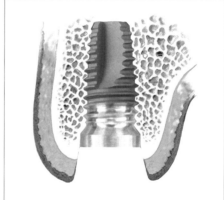

Fig 9-3 Implant with healing abutment removed.

The entire implant platform should be visible. If there is any soft tissue over the surface (Fig 9-4), this should be carefully removed with a plastic- or gold-tipped scaler to avoid damaging the implant surface.

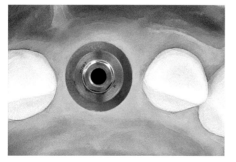 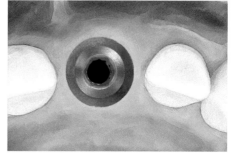

Fig 9-4 Ensure that there is no soft tissue obscuring the implant platform.

external	internal

To ascertain the height of the collar that is required for the abutment, measure the height of the soft tissue using either a periodontal probe (Fig 9-5) or a tissue measuring post.

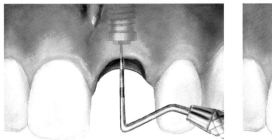 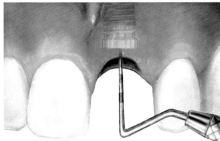

Fig 9-5 Use of a periodontal probe to measure the height of tissue above the implant.

Select the abutment height that best fits the tooth that is being replaced. As a guide, the collar of the abutment should lie approximately 1 mm below the gingival margin. Place the abutment over the head of the implant (Fig 9-6). Rotate the abutment slightly to ensure the hexagon on the underside of the abutment fully engages the hexagon of the implant.

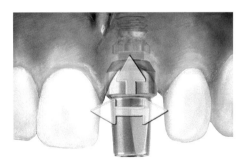 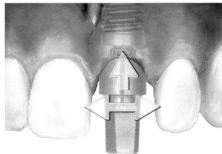

Fig 9-6 Placement of abutment to engage the hex of the implant. When seated, the prepared finish line on the abutment should be about 1 mm below the soft tissue at the highest point (usually interproximally).

Take the hexed try-in screw and use the hex driver to initially tighten the screw and secure the abutment to the implant (Fig 9-7).

| external | internal |

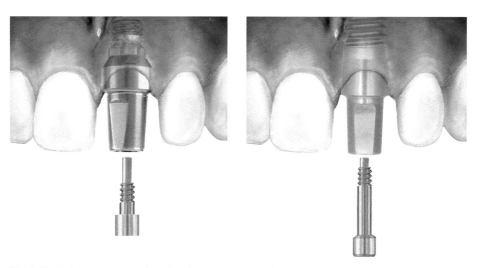

Fig 9-7 Try-in screw securing the abutment to the implant.

A long cone radiograph is taken to verify that the abutment is fully seated on the head of the implant (Fig 9-8). If a space is evident *(left of each frame)*, loosen the screw and rotate the abutment slightly until it feels locked into place *(right of each frame)*. Retighten the screw and retake the radiograph if necessary.

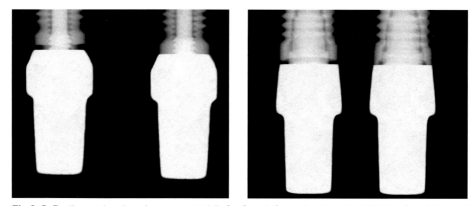

Fig 9-8 Radiographs showing unseated *(left of each frame)* and seated *(right of each frame)* abutments on the implants.

The abutment is then prepared following normal restorative procedures (Fig 9-9), ensuring that the correct retention and resistance forms are achieved. To avoid over-preparation of the abutment, it is recommended that the hand piece is operated at 40,000 rpm. Copious water spray is required to prevent overheating the implant.

external	internal

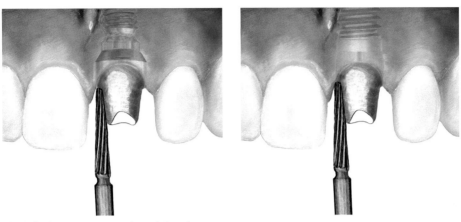

Fig 9-9 Outline preparation of the abutment.

The abutment is prepared using the following burs:
- H33L.31.021 (Brasseler) for gross cutting in combination with 703L.FG (tapered fissure bur)
- H158.31.012 H297FG, which is a carbide finishing bur for final refinement of the abutment.

Refinement of the abutment preparation can be completed outside the mouth (Fig 9-10) using an abutment holder. Fine stones and rubber wheels may be used to achieve a smooth finish.

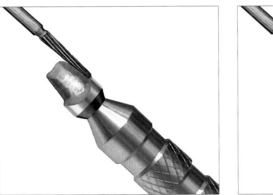 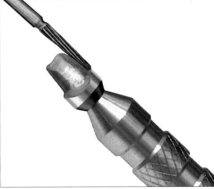

Fig 9-10 Refinement of a preparation outside the mouth.

The abutment is returned to the implant and secured with the appropriate permanent screw and driver (Fig 9-11). A square screw may be used to attach the abutment to the external hex implant as it can achieve a higher preload. A hexed screw is used to attach the abutment to the internal connection implant.

external	internal

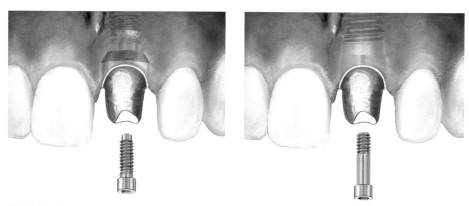

Fig 9-11 Securing the abutment with a permanent screw.

A long cone radiograph is taken to verify that the prepared abutment is fully down on to the head of the implant (Fig 9-12). If a space is evident *(left of each frame)*, loosen the screw and rotate the abutment slightly until it feels locked into place *(right of each frame)*. Re-tighten the screw and retake the radiograph if necessary. Check abutment preparation and make any final adjustments (Fig 9-13).

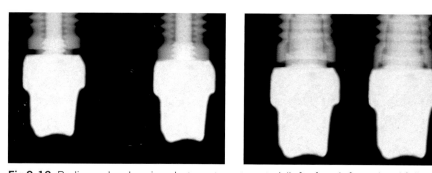

Fig 9-12 Radiographs showing abutments not seated *(left of each frame)* and fully seated *(right of each frame)*.

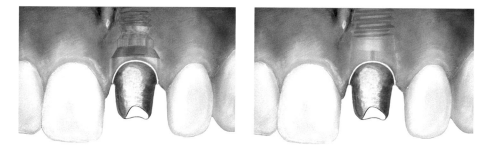

Fig 9-13 Checking the abutment preparation and making any final adjustments.

external	internal

As a guide, a 5–7 degree taper should be achieved on the axial walls. The facial finish line should be a smooth chamfer, 1 mm subgingival, and follow the natural contours of the gingival tissue.

The square-ended driver tip (external hex implant) or hex-ended driver tip (internal connection implant) is placed in the restorative torque indicator (Fig 9-14). The screw is tightened using the indicator to 35 Ncm (square screw) or 20 Ncm (hex screw).

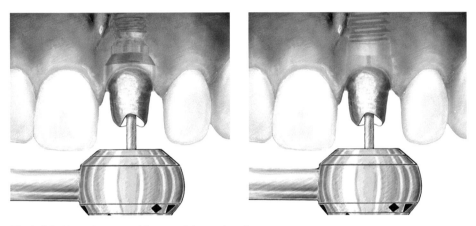

Fig 9-14 Use of torque driver to tighten the abutment screw.

The restorative torque indicator is rotated clockwise until the triangle on the inner ring and the diamond on the outer ring are coincident; this gives a torque of 35 Ncm (for a square screw) (Fig 9-15a). When the triangle on the inner ring and the triangle on the outer ring are coincident, the torque is 20 Ncm (for a hex screw) (Fig 9-15b).

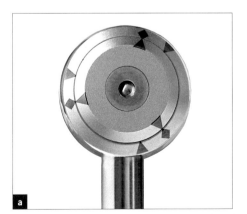
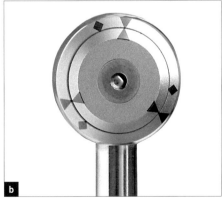

Fig 9-15 Restorative torque indicator showing marks for the application of different torque to screws. Triangle on the inner ring aligned with the diamond on the outer ring gives 35 Ncm torque (a), and aligned with the triangle on the outer ring gives 20 Ncm torque (b).

external	internal

The access hole is first filled with silicone material or polytetrafluoroethylene (PTFE; Teflon) tape followed by an intermediate restorative material. This ensures that when the final impression is made the material will not enter the screw hole and cause distortion of the impression.

Retraction cord is placed into the gingival sulcus. This retracts the tissue to enable the operator to see the entire finish line prior to making an impression, and also allows any further minor adjustments to the abutment to be made. Once retraction of the tissue has been achieved, an impression is made using a material of the operator's choice (Fig 9-16). An opposing impression is made together with an interocclusal record and shade prescription for the laboratory technician (Fig 9-17).

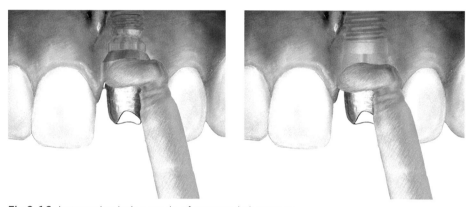

Fig 9-16 Impression being made of prepared abutment.

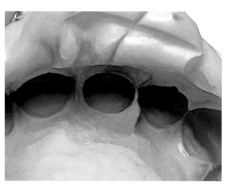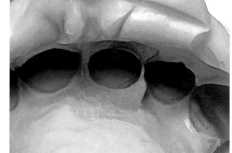

Fig 9-17 Impression of prepared abutment.

A provisional restoration may be constructed using a pre-formed crown, relined with a resin material (Fig 9-18). Once this material has set, it can be adjusted, polished, and then cemented onto the abutment with a temporary cement.

external	internal

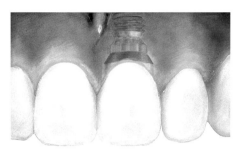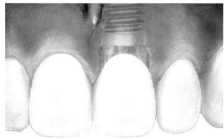

Fig 9-18 Provisional crown in place on the prepared abutment.

In the laboratory, a die is prepared from the impression to construct the final restoration (Figs 9-19 and 9-20). The restoration is then returned to the clinician, ready for insertion.

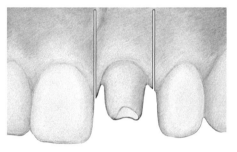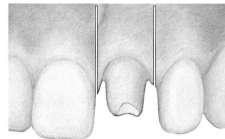

Fig 9-19 Preparing dies for the definitive crown.

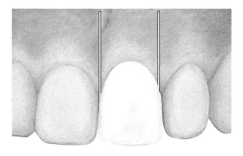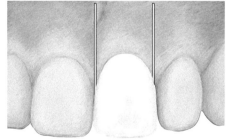

Fig 9-20 Completed crown on the die.

external	internal

The restoration is then tried in the mouth to check shade, contour, and occlusion. It is then cemented over the abutment using either temporary or long-term cement (Fig 9-21). Temporary cement allows for the possibility of retrieving the restoration if the abutment screw becomes loose.

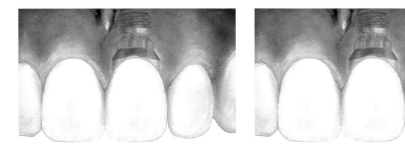

Fig 9-21 Final restoration checked and cemented on the implant abutment.

Alternatively, the abutment may be prepared immediately following second-stage surgery. A provisional crown is placed on the abutment for the healing period (6–8 weeks). At the next visit, the abutment preparation may be refined to accommodate soft tissue changes that may have occurred. The impression of the abutment is made and the crown completed as described.

CHAPTER 10

Single-tooth Restoration Using an Indirect Technique with a Preparable Abutment

| external | | internal |

Materials and components

- hexagonal driver
- square driver
- impression tray
- impression coping with guide pin
- adhesive
- impression material

- restorative torque indicator with square or hexed driver tip
- occlusal registration material
- locking tweezers
- cement material

Procedure

At second-stage implant surgery, a flared healing abutment is placed on the implant and the tissues are allowed to heal for 6 to 8 weeks. The healing abutment should be visible at least 1 mm above the level of the soft tissue (Fig 10-1).

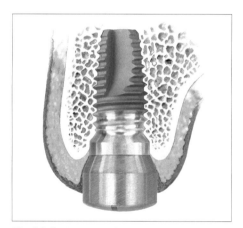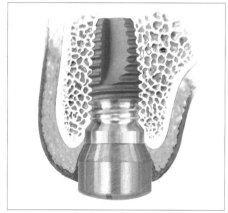

Fig 10-1 Implant after healing period at second-stage surgery with healing abutment in place.

The provisional denture or fixed partial denture is removed and set aside. The provisional healing abutment is unscrewed using a hexagonal screwdriver (Figs 10-2 and 10-3). It is useful to place a square of gauze behind the operating area as the components are quite small and it prevents possible loss of the abutment if the patient swallows.

external	internal

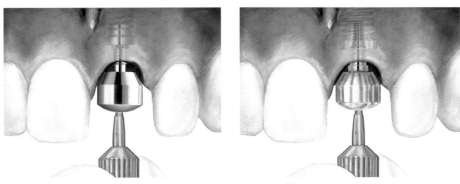

Fig 10-2 Healing abutment removed using hexagonal driver.

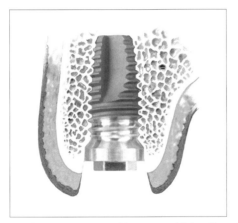 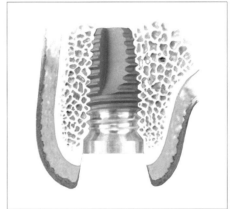

Fig 10-3 Side view of implant with healing abutment removed.

The entire implant platform should be visible. If there is any soft tissue over the surface, this should be carefully removed with a plastic- or gold-tipped scaler to avoid damaging the implant surface (Fig 10-4).

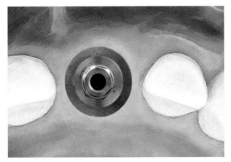 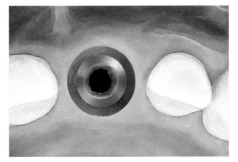

Fig 10-4 Ensure that there is no soft tissue obscuring the top of the implant.

external	internal

An implant impression coping and guide pin are placed on the implant and the fitting surfaces of the implant and the impression coping are aligned (Fig 10-5).

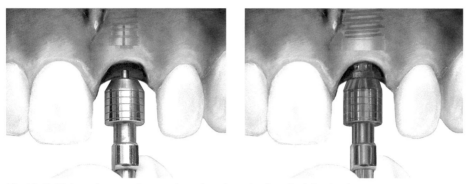

Fig 10-5 Pick-up impression coping placed on the head of the implant.

The impression coping guide pin is then hand tightened and secured using a hexagonal driver (Fig 10-6).

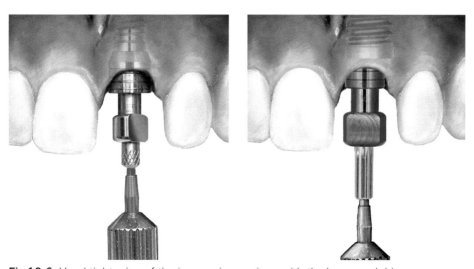

Fig 10-6 Hand tightening of the impression copings with the hexagonal driver.

159

external	internal

It is important to ensure that the impression coping assembly is fully seated on the implant. Usually this cannot be verified directly, and a long cone periapical radiograph should be taken (Fig 10-7). If a space is evident (*left of each frame*), loosen the guide pin and rotate the impression coping slightly until it feels locked into place (*right of each frame*). Retighten the guide pin and retake the radiograph if necessary.

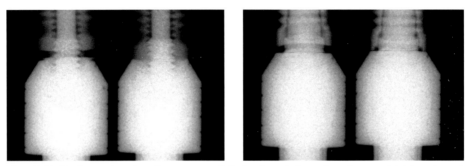

Fig 10-7 Radiographs showing unseated *(left of each frame)* and seated *(right of each frame)* abutments on the implants.

A hole is made in the impression tray and the tray is tried in to ensure that the guide pin protrudes through the opening (Fig 10-8). The impression tray is then uniformly coated with a thin layer of adhesive, corresponding to the impression material that is going to be used, and allowed to dry.

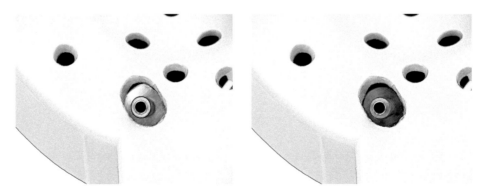

Fig 10-8 Open tray with impression coping guide pin showing through.

external	internal

The tray can then be filled with impression material. While the tray is being loaded, a light-bodied impression material is carefully syringed around the impression coping and the surrounding soft tissue (Fig 10-9). This is essential, as it allows the laboratory technician to produce a cast that has an accurate duplication of the soft tissue surrounding the implant. An accurate impression of the tissue will allow the technician to create the final restoration with the correct emergence profile.

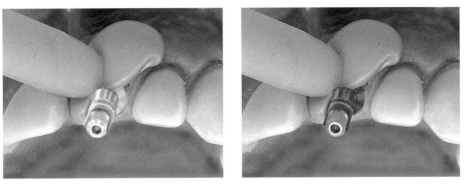

Fig 10-9 Impression material syringed around the impression coping.

The filled tray is then inserted into the mouth, ensuring that the guide pin is visible and protrudes through the hole in the custom tray (Fig 10-10).

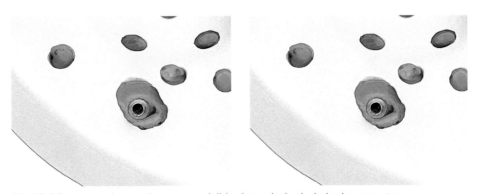

Fig 10-10 Impression coping screw visible through the hole in the open tray.

external	internal

When the material has set, the impression coping pin is unscrewed using a hexagonal driver (Fig 10-11). It is essential that the pin is fully disengaged from the implant before the impression is removed from the mouth.

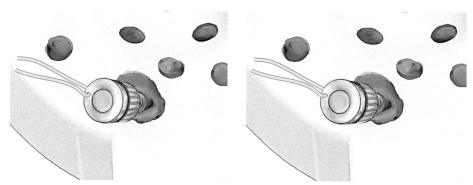

Fig 10-11 Disengaging the impression coping from the implant.

Disengagement of the guide pin is verified by gently lifting the pin with a pair of locking tweezers (Fig 10-12). The pin should move freely without resistance.

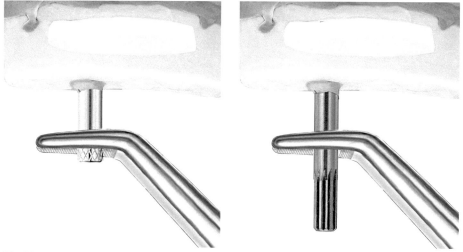

Fig 10-12 Checking the impression coping pin is disengaged.

external	internal

The impression can then be removed from the mouth and disinfected prior to sending it to the laboratory technician (Fig 10-13). It is important to check that the impression coping is firmly embedded in the impression so that no movement of the coping is evident. If the coping moves in the impression, the procedure should be repeated.

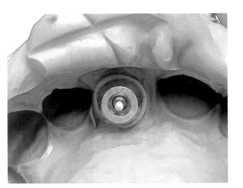 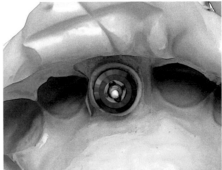

Fig 10-13 Completed impression removed from the mouth.

The healing abutment is then replaced and tightened using a hexagonal driver (Fig 10-14). It is essential that the abutment is fully down onto the implant to ensure that no soft tissue can spread over the head of the implant. An opposing impression is made together with an interocclusal record and shade prescription for the laboratory technician. The patient's provisional restoration should be checked and replaced.

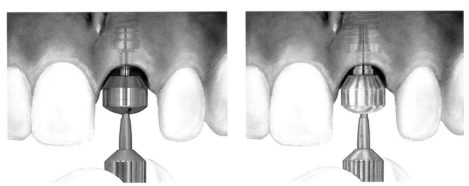

Fig 10-14 Replacing the healing abutment on the implant after removal of the impression.

external	internal

The laboratory returns the prepared abutment, the locating jig, the try-in screw, the final abutment screw, and the definitive restoration (Fig 10-15).

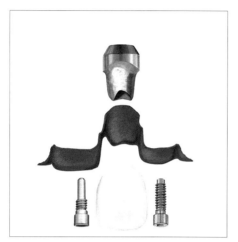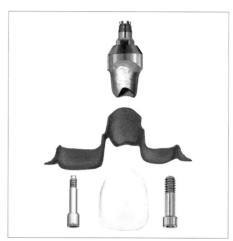

Fig 10-15 The restoration and components returned from the laboratory.

It is important that the abutment can be correctly orientated when finally screwed down on to the head of the implant. This is achieved by the construction of a locating jig (Fig 10-16). The jig is made in the laboratory, using a quick-cure laboratory resin, after the abutment has been prepared by the technician.

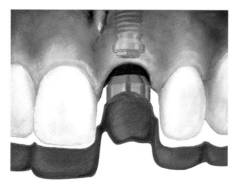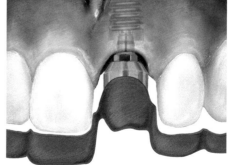

Fig 10-16 Use of locating jig to correctly orientate the abutment on the implant.

external	internal

The jig should fit accurately over the prepared abutment and should also locate over the adjacent teeth to provide stability (Fig 10-17). The jig securely holds the abutment in place while the try-in screw is tightened using a hexed driver.

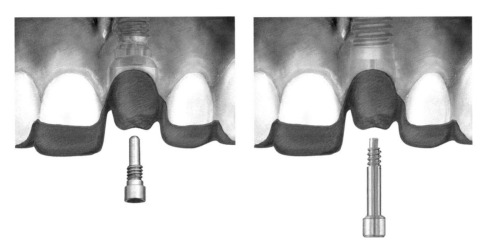

Fig 10-17 Locating jig holding the abutment on the implant to allow screw placement.

Take a long cone radiograph to verify that the prepared abutment is fully down onto the head of the implant (Fig 10-18). If a space is evident (*left of each frame*), the master cast is inaccurate and the impression must be retaken.

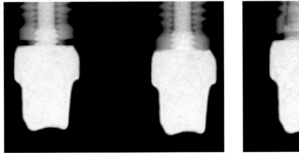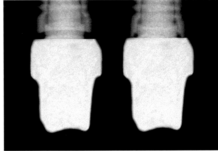

Fig 10-18 Radiographs to verify full seating of the abutment.

external	internal

Once the seating of the abutment has been verified radiographically, the locating jig is removed leaving the prepared abutment in place (Fig 10-19). The final restoration is then tried in the mouth to verify the contour, aesthetics, function, and occlusion (Fig 10-20).

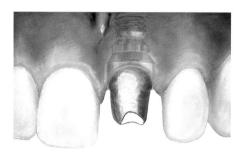 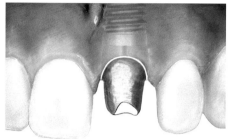

Fig 10-19 Prepared abutment in position.

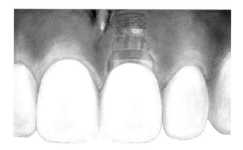 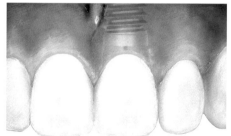

Fig 10-20 Try-in of final restoration.

When the operator is satisfied with the restoration, it is removed and the locating jig is repositioned on the abutment. The try-in screw is then removed and replaced with the final abutment screw, which is hand tightened with the driver (Fig 10-21). For an external hex implant, a square-headed screw may be used, whereas a hexagonal screw is placed on the internal connection implant.

external	internal

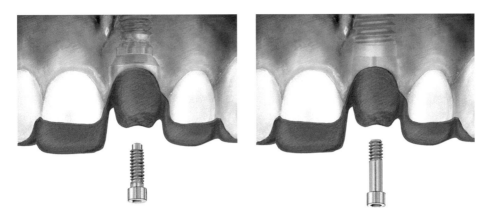

Fig 10-21 Verified abutment ready to be screwed in place.

The square-ended driver tip (external hex implant) or hex-ended driver tip (internal connection implant) is placed in the restorative torque indicator. The screw is tightened the correct amount using the restorative torque indicator (Fig 10-22).

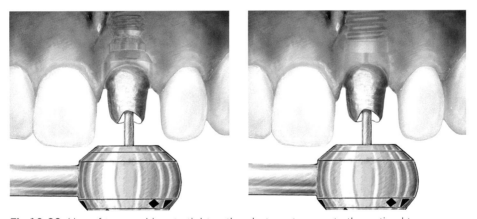

Fig 10-22 Use of torque driver to tighten the abutment screw to the optimal torque.

The restorative torque indicator is rotated clockwise until the triangle on the inner ring and the diamond on the outer ring are coincident. This gives a torque of 35 Ncm (external hex) (Fig 10-23a). When the triangle on the inner ring and the triangle on the outer ring are coincident, the torque is 20 Ncm (internal connection) (Fig 10-23b).

external   internal

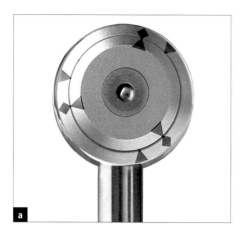 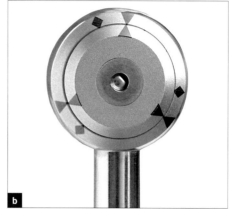

Fig 10-23 Restorative torque indicator showing marks for the application of different torque to screws. Triangle on the inner ring aligned with the diamond on the outer ring gives 35 Ncm torque (a), and aligned with the triangle on the outer ring gives 20 Ncm torque (b).

The restoration is then tried in the mouth to check shade, contour, and occlusion. It is then cemented over the abutment using either temporary or long-term cement (Fig 10-24). Temporary cement allows the possibility of retrieving the restoration if the abutment screw becomes loose.

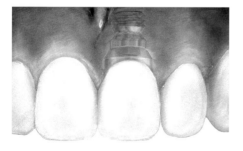 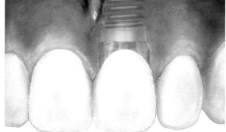

Fig 10-24 Crown cemented in place.

Cemented Single-tooth Restoration Using a UCLA Abutment

external	internal

Materials and components

- hexagonal driver
- square driver
- impression tray
- impression coping with guide pin
- adhesive
- impression material

- restorative torque indicator with square or hexed driver tip
- occlusal registration material
- locking tweezers
- cement material

Procedure

At second-stage implant surgery, a flared healing abutment is placed on the implant and the tissues are allowed to heal for 6–8 weeks. The healing abutment should be visible at least 1 mm above the level of the soft tissue (Fig 11-1).

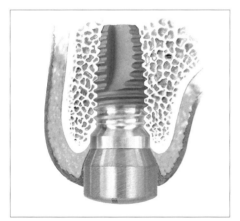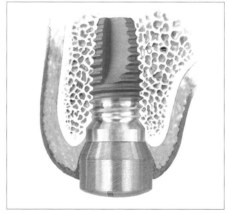

Fig 11-1 Implant after healing period at second-stage surgery with healing abutment in place.

The provisional denture or fixed partial denture is removed and set aside. Remove the provisional healing abutment that has been in place using a hexagonal screwdriver (Figs 11-2 and 11-3). It is useful to place a square of gauze behind the operating area as the components are quite small, and this prevents possible loss of the abutment if the patient swallows.

| external | internal |

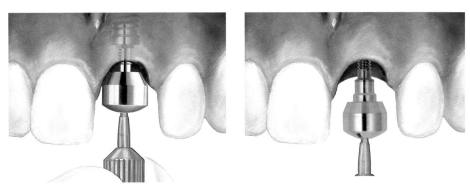

Fig 11-2 Healing abutment removed using hexagonal driver.

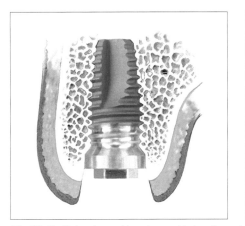 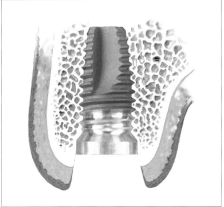

Fig 11-3 Side view of implant with healing abutment removed.

The entire implant platform should be visible. If there is any soft tissue over the surface, this should be carefully removed with a plastic- or gold-tipped scaler to avoid damaging the implant surface (Fig 11-4).

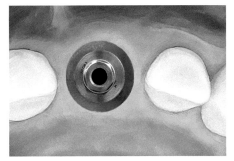 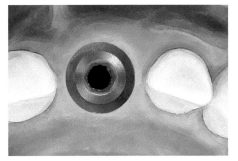

Fig 11-4 Ensure that there is no soft tissue obscuring the implant platform.

external	internal

An implant impression coping and guide pin are placed on the implant, and the hexagons of the implant and the impression coping are aligned (Fig 11-5).The guide pin is then hand tightened and finally secured using a hexagonal driver (Fig 11-6).

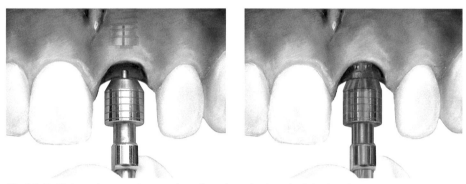

Fig 11-5 Pick-up impression coping placed on the head of the implant.

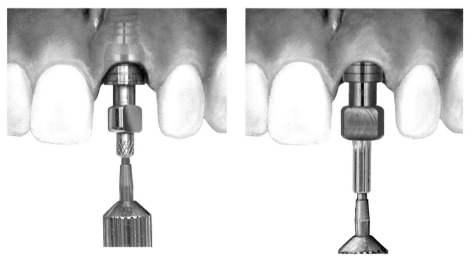

Fig 11-6 Hand tightening of the impression copings with the hexagonal driver.

It is important to ensure that the impression coping assembly is fully seated on the implant. Usually this cannot be verified directly, and a long cone periapical radiograph should be taken (Fig 11-7). If a space is evident (*left of each frame*), loosen the guide pin and slightly rotate the impression coping until it feels locked into place (*right of each frame*). Retighten the guide pin and retake the radiograph if necessary.

| external | internal |

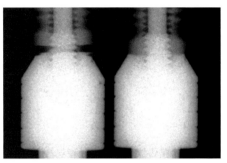 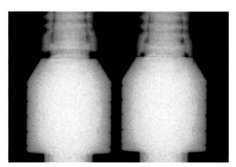

Fig 11-7 Radiographs showing unseated *(left of each frame)* and seated *(right of each frame)* impression copings on the implants.

A hole is made in the impression tray and the tray is tried in to ensure that the guide pin protrudes through the opening (Fig 11-8). The impression tray is then uniformly coated with a thin layer of adhesive, corresponding to the impression material that is going to be used, and allowed to dry.

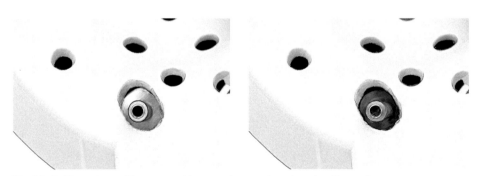

Fig 11-8 Open tray with screw of impression coping showing through.

The tray can then be filled with impression material. While the tray is being loaded, impression material is carefully syringed around the impression coping and the surrounding soft tissue (Fig 11-9). This is essential, as it allows the laboratory technician to produce a cast that has an accurate duplication of the soft tissue surrounding the implant. An accurate impression of the tissue will allow the technician to create the final restoration with the correct emergence profile.

external	internal

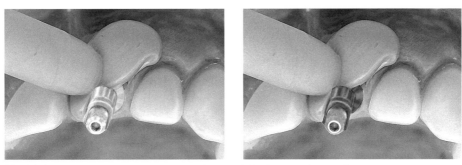

Fig 11-9 Impression material syringed around the impression coping.

The filled tray is then inserted into the mouth, ensuring that the guide pin is visible and protrudes through the hole in the custom tray (Fig 11-10).

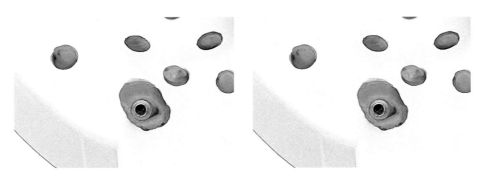

Fig 11-10 Impression coping screw visible through the hole in the open tray.

When the material has set, the impression coping pin is unscrewed using a hexagonal driver (Fig 11-11). It is essential that the pin be fully disengaged from the implant before the impression is removed from the mouth.

external	internal

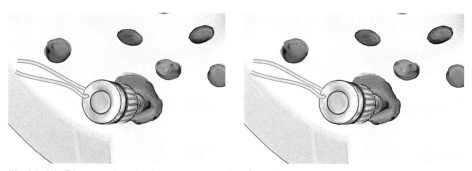

Fig 11-11 Disengaging the impression coping from the implant

Disengagement of the guide pin is verified by gently lifting the pin with a pair of locking tweezers (Fig 11-12). The pin should move freely without resistance.

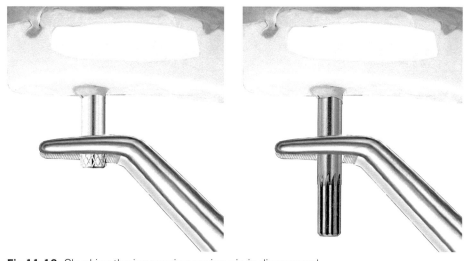

Fig 11-12 Checking the impression coping pin is disengaged.

The impression can then be removed from the mouth and disinfected prior to sending it to the laboratory technician (Fig 11-13). It is essential to check that the impression coping is firmly embedded in the impression so no movement of the coping is evident. If the coping moves in the impression, the procedure should be repeated.

| external | internal |

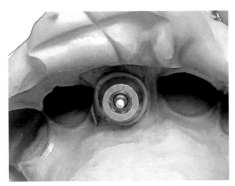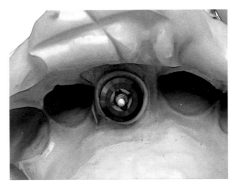

Fig 11-13 Completed impression removed from the mouth.

The healing abutment is then replaced and tightened using a hexagonal driver (Fig 11-14). It is essential that the abutment be fully screwed down onto the implant to ensure that no soft tissue will proliferate over the head of the implant. An opposing impression is made together with an interocclusal record and shade prescription for the laboratory technician. The patient's provisional restoration should be checked and replaced.

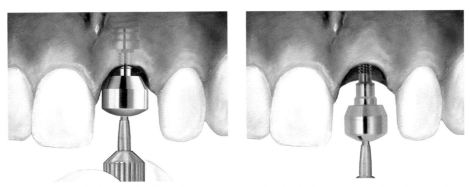

Fig 11-14 Replacing the healing abutment on the implant after removal of the impression.

The laboratory returns the completed UCLA abutment, the locating jig, the try-in screw, the final abutment screw, and the definitive restoration for try-in (Fig 11-15).

external	internal

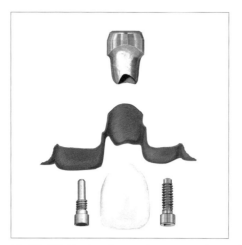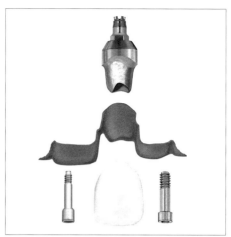

Fig 11-15 Restoration and components ready for try-in.

It is important that the UCLA abutment can be correctly orientated when finally screwed down on to the head of the implant. This is achieved by the construction of a locating jig (Fig 11-16). The jig is made in the laboratory, using a quick-cure laboratory resin, after the abutment has been completed by the technician.

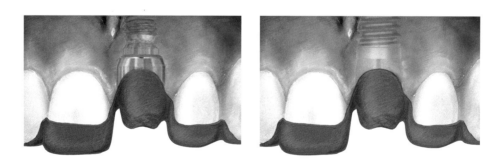

Fig 11-16 Locating jig used to seat the cast UCLA abutment on the implant.

The jig should fit accurately over the UCLA abutment and should also locate over the adjacent teeth to provide stability. The jig securely holds the abutment in place while the try-in screw is tightened using a hexed driver (Fig 11-17).

external	internal

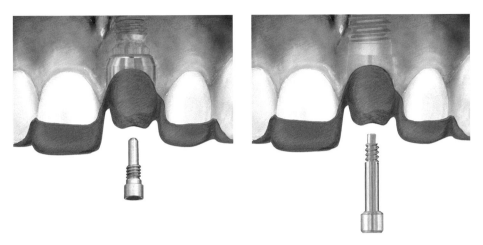

Fig 11-17 Try-in screw used to secure the UCLA abutment.

A long cone radiograph is taken to verify that the UCLA abutment is fully down onto the head of the implant (Fig 11-18). If a space is evident (*left of each frame*), the master cast is inaccurate and, therefore, the impression must be retaken. A fully seated abutment is shown on the right of each frame.

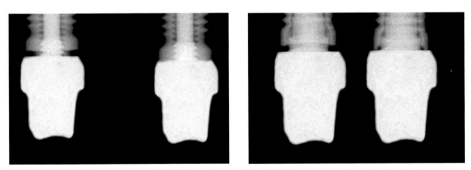

Fig 11-18 Radiograph to verify full seating of the UCLA abutment on the implant.

Once the seating of the UCLA abutment has been verified radiographically, the locating jig is removed leaving the abutment on the implant (Fig 11-19).

external	internal

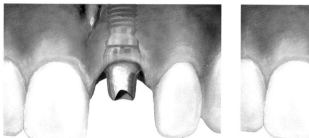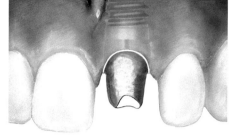

Fig 11-19 Verified UCLA abutment on the implant.

The definitive restoration is then tried in the mouth to verify the contour, aesthetics, function, and occlusion (Fig 11-20).

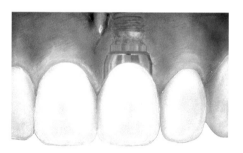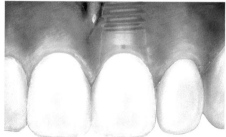

Fig 11-20 Try-in of definitive restoration on the abutment.

When the restoration is verified, it is removed and the locating jig is repositioned over the UCLA abutment. The try-in screw is then removed and replaced with the final abutment screw, which is tightened by hand with the driver (Fig 11-21). A square-headed screw may be used on the external hex implant, while a hexed screw is used on the internal connection implant.

external	internal

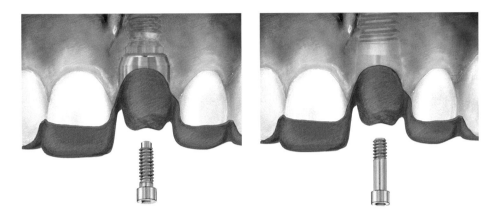

Fig 11-21 Placement of final screw to secure the UCLA abutment.

The driver tip is placed into the restorative torque indicator (Fig 11-22). The square screw (external hex implant) is tightened to 35 Ncm, while the hexed screw (internal connection implant) is tightened to 20 Ncm. The restorative torque indicator is rotated clockwise until the triangle on the inner ring and the diamond on the outer ring are coincident; this gives a torque of 35 Ncm (for external hex implant) (Fig 11-23a). When the triangle on the inner ring and the triangle on the outer ring are coincident, the torque is 20 Ncm (for internal connection implant) (Fig 11-23b).

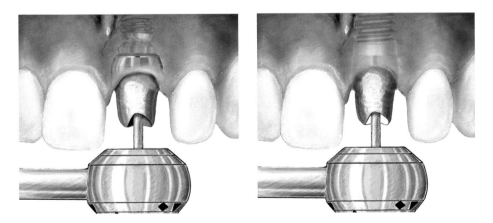

Fig 11-22 Use of torque driver to tighten the abutment screw to the optimal torque.

| external | internal |

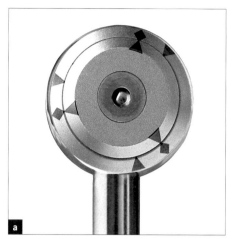 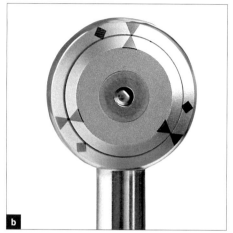

Fig 11-23 Use of torque indicator to apply the correct preload to the abutment screw. The triangle on the inner ring aligned with the diamond on the outer ring gives 35 Ncm torque (a), and aligned with the triangle on the outer ring gives 20 Ncm torque (b).

The screw access hole in the abutment is sealed with silicone material, wax, or PTFE tape. The crown is then cemented over the abutment using either temporary or long-term cement (Fig 11-24). Temporary cement allows the restoration to be retrieved more easily if the abutment screw becomes loose.

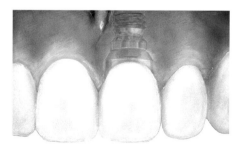 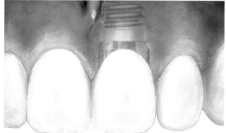

Fig 11-24 Definitive crown cemented on the tightened abutment.

Screw-retained Single Restoration Using a Conical Abutment

external	internal

Material and components required

- hexagonal driver
- impression tray
- impression material
- periodontal probe or measuring post
- impression coping with guide pin
- restorative torque indicator with conical abutment driver tip

- abutment hand driver
- occlusal registration material
- cement material
- gauze square
- retaining screw

Procedure

Remove the provisional healing abutment using a hexagonal screwdriver (Figs 12-1 and 12–2). It is useful to place a square of gauze behind the operating area, as the components are quite small and this prevents possible loss of the abutment if the patient swallows.

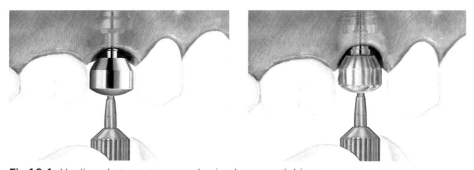

Fig 12-1 Healing abutment removed using hexagonal driver.

external	internal

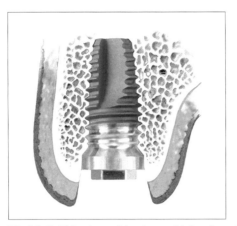 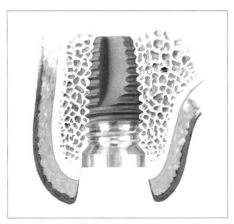

Fig 12-2 Side view of implant with healing abutment removed.

The entire implant platform should be visible. If there is any soft tissue over the surface, this should be carefully removed with a plastic- or gold-tipped scaler to avoid damaging the implant surface (Fig 12-3).

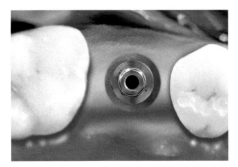 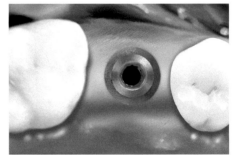

Fig 12-3 Ensure that there is no soft tissue obscuring the implant platform.

To ascertain the height of the collar that is required for the conical abutment, measure the height of the soft tissue using either a periodontal probe (Fig 12-4) or a tissue measuring post. As a guide, the collar of the conical abutment should lie approximately 1 mm below the gingival margin.

external	internal

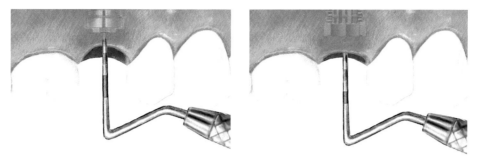

Fig 12-4 Use of a periodontal probe to measure the height of tissue above the implant.

The conical abutment is removed from the sterilizing pouch and is supplied with an integral disposable driver (Fig 12-5). The abutment is a two-piece unit consisting of a collar that engages the hexagon of the implant and a screw that secures the abutment to the implant (Fig 12-6).

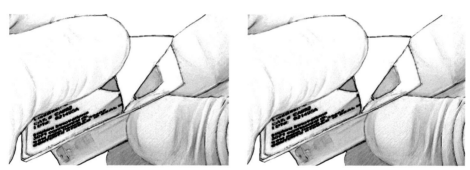

Fig 12-5 Hand tightening of conical abutment impression coping with hex driver.

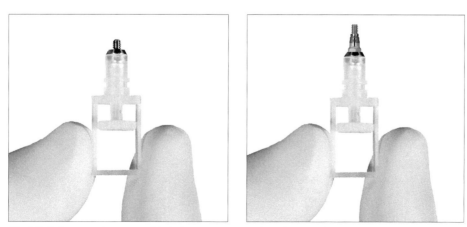

Fig 12-6 Impression tray with hole to accommodate impression coping guide pin.

The collar of the abutment is located over the head of the implant and fully seated to engage the hex (Fig 12-7). It is possible to feel the abutment seated fully on the implant.

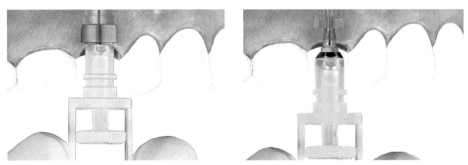

Fig 12-7 Seating the conical abutment on to the head of the implant.

Once the collar is fully seated, the central screw is tightened down manually via the plastic driver (Fig 12-8).The disposable driver can now be removed from the abutment leaving the secured abutment in place (Fig 12-9).

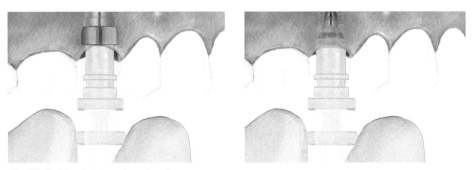

Fig 12-8 Hand tightening the abutment screw.

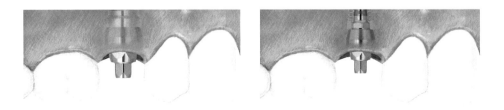

Fig 12-9 Secured conical abutment in place.

The seating of the conical abutment collar on the implant is verified using a long cone radiograph (Fig 12-10). If the abutment is not seated fully, then the central abutment screw should be loosened slightly and the abutment rotated until it engages the head of the implant.

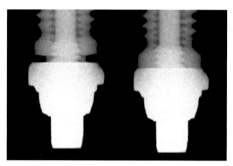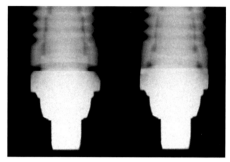

Fig 12-10 Radiograph showing conical abutment not fully seated *(left of each frame)* and completely seated *(right of each frame)*.

The conical abutment is hand tightened using an abutment driver that is designed to fit over the abutment screw (Fig 12-11).

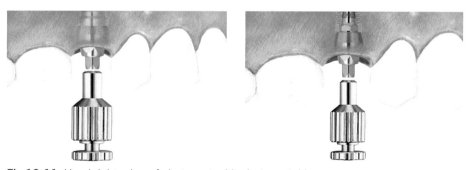

Fig 12-11 Hand tightening of abutment with abutment driver.

The conical abutment driver tip is placed into the restorative torque indicator (Fig 12-12). The screws are tightened to 20 Ncm using the indicator. The restorative torque indicator is rotated clockwise until the triangle on the inner ring and the triangle on the outer ring are coincident (Fig 12-13). At that point, 20 Ncm torque has been achieved.

external	internal

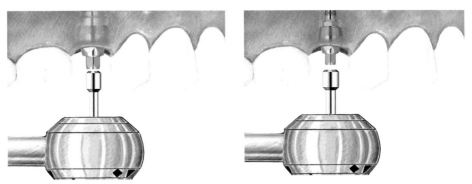

Fig 12-12 Use of abutment driver with the restorative torque indicator to tighten the abutment screw.

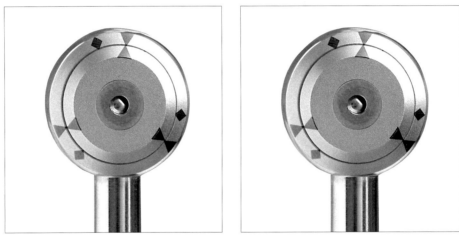

Fig 12-13 Restorative torque indicator showing marks for the application of different torques. The triangle on the inner ring aligned with the triangle on the outer ring gives 20 Ncm torque.

For single-unit restorations, the impression coping with an internal hexagon must be selected (Fig 12-14). This type of impression coping records the position of the hexagon on the conical abutment. Recording the hexagon prevents the restoration from rotating around the abutment.

external	internal

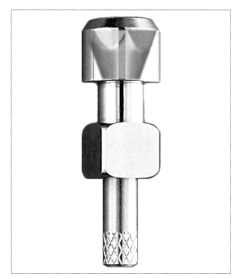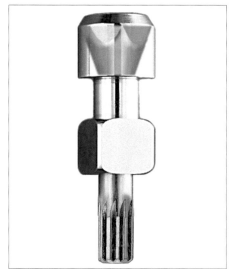

Fig 12-14 Conical abutment impression copings.

The impression coping is placed over the abutment and the guide pin tightened using a hexagonal driver (Fig 12-15). It is important to remember that the impression coping fits over the conical abutment and not directly on the head of the implant.

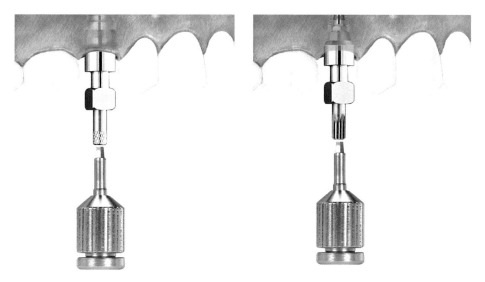

Fig 12-15 Hand tightening of conical abutment impression coping with hex driver.

It is essential to verify that the impression coping assembly is fully seated on the abutment. Usually this is possible to do directly, but if this is not the case, a long cone periapical radiograph will be required.

A hole is made in the impression tray and the tray is tried in to ensure that the impression coping guide pin protrudes through the opening (Fig 12-16). The tray is then removed from the mouth and uniformly coated with a thin layer of adhesive, corresponding to the impression material that is going to be used, and allowed to dry.

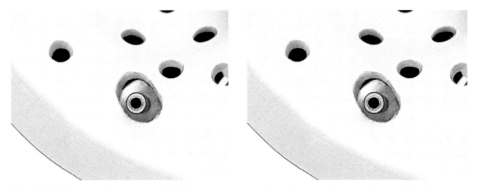

Fig 12-16 Impression tray with hole to accommodate impression coping guide pin.

The tray can then be filled with impression material. While the tray is being loaded, impression material is carefully syringed around the impression coping and the surrounding soft tissue (Fig 12-17). This is essential, as it allows the laboratory technician to produce a cast that has an accurate duplication of the soft tissue surrounding the implant. An accurate impression of the tissue will allow the technician to create the final restoration with the correct emergence profile.

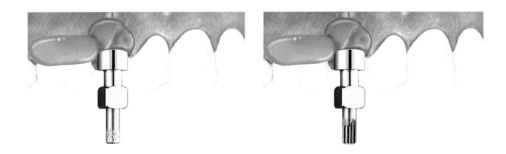

Fig 12-17 Impression material syringed around impression coping and teeth.

external	internal

The filled tray is then inserted into the mouth, ensuring that the impression coping pin is visible and protruding through the hole in the impression tray (Fig 12-18).

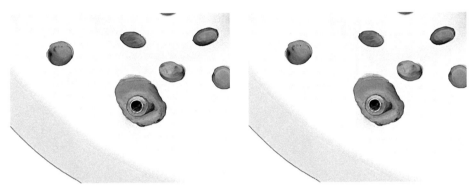

Fig 12-18 Impression tray seated with impression coping guide pin visible.

When the material has set, the impression coping pin is unscrewed from the abutment using a hexagonal driver (Fig 12-19).

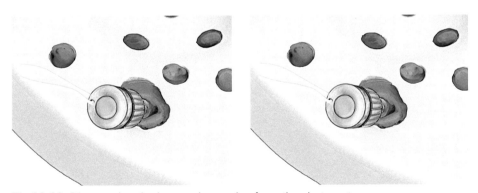

Fig 12-19 Disengaging the impression coping from the abutment.

Check that the guide pin is disengaged from the abutment by gently sliding it away with locking tweezers (Fig 12-20).

external	internal

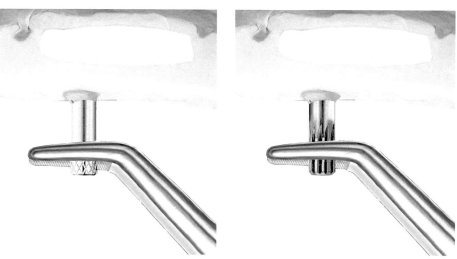

Fig 12-20 Checking the impression coping pin is disengaged.

The impression can then be removed from the mouth and disinfected prior to sending it to the laboratory. It is essential to check that the impression coping is firmly embedded in the impression so that no movement of the coping is evident (Fig 12-21). If the coping moves in the impression, the procedure should be repeated.

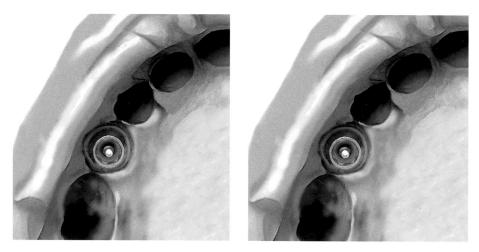

Fig 12-21 Completed impression with coping securely in place.

external	internal

A provisional cap is placed and tightened using a hexagonal driver (Fig 12-22). It is essential that the cap be fully seated down on to the conical abutment to ensure that no soft tissue will proliferate between the components. An opposing impression is made together with an interocclusal record and shade prescription for the laboratory technician. If the patient has a provisional restoration, it should be checked and reinserted.

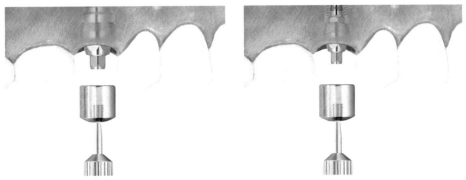

Fig 12-22 Placing the provisional cap on the conical abutment.

Once the definitive crown is returned from the laboratory, the provisional cap is removed. The crown is tried in to verify fit, contour, occlusion, and aesthetics (Fig 12-23).

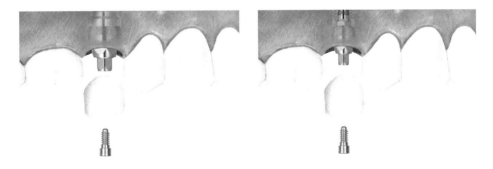

Fig 12-23 Try-in of crown using the retaining screw.

external	internal

The retaining screw is tightened using a hexagonal driver. The recommended torque for the retaining screw is 10 Ncm, which can be achieved by hand tightening (Fig 12-24). It is essential that a small square of gauze is placed behind the crown to ensure the patient does not accidentally swallow the small retaining screw.

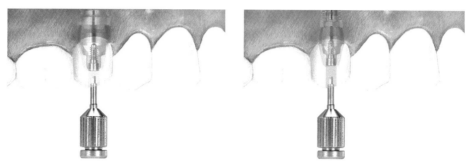

Fig 12-24 Tightening the small retaining screw with a hand driver.

The access hole is temporarily filled with a small pledget of cotton wool at the base and covered with an intermediate restorative material. The patient is recalled after 1 week and the intermediate restorative material and cotton wool are removed. The tightness of the retaining screw is verified and the access hole filled with silicone material or PTFE tape at the base, and at least 2 mm of resin composite on the occlusal surface (Fig 12-25).

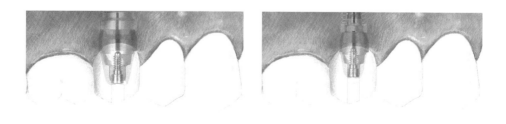

Fig 12-25 Definitive crown in place with screw access hole sealed.

CHAPTER 13

Single-unit Alternative Impression Technique Using Transfer Copings (Closed-tray Technique)

external	internal

An alternative impression technique is available using transfer impression copings that are designed to remain screwed on to the implant or an abutment (e.g. conical abutment) when the impression is removed from the mouth. In this case, access holes for the transfer copings are not required in the impression tray. The transfer coping consists of a central screw that secures an outer cylinder to the implant or abutment. The technique may be used for single- or multi-unit restorations.

The advantages of the transfer coping are that it can be used where there is limited space for a driver and trimming of the impression tray is not required, hence simplifying the procedure. The disadvantage of this technique is that the transfer copings must be repositioned in the impression after it is removed from the mouth. It is sometimes difficult to correctly place the transfer copings in the impression, which will lead to an inaccurate master cast.

Procedure

Remove the provisional healing abutment using a hexagonal screwdriver (Figs 13-1 and Fig 13-2). It is useful to place a square of gauze behind the operating area, as the components are quite small and this prevents possible loss of the abutment if the patient swallows.

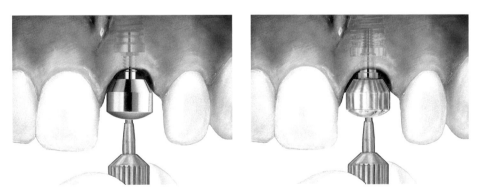

Fig 13-1 Use of hexagonal driver to remove the healing abutment.

external	internal

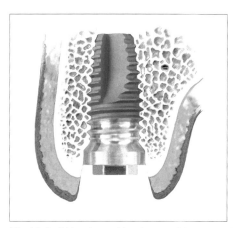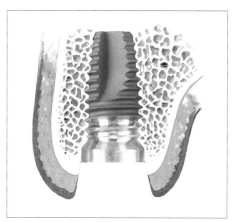

Fig 13-2 Side view of implants with the healing abutment removed.

The entire implant platform should be visible. If there is any soft tissue over the surface, this should be carefully removed with a plastic- or gold-tipped scaler to avoid damaging the implant surface (Fig 13-3).

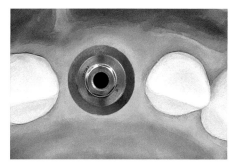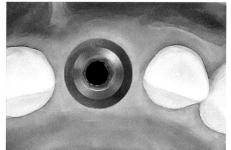

Fig 13-3 Ensure that there is no soft tissue obscuring the implant platform.

Transfer copings are placed on the implant, taking care that the copings align with the external hex or internal connection of the implant (Fig 13-4). The transfer coping is finger tightened and checked for stability on the implant (Fig 13-5).

external	internal

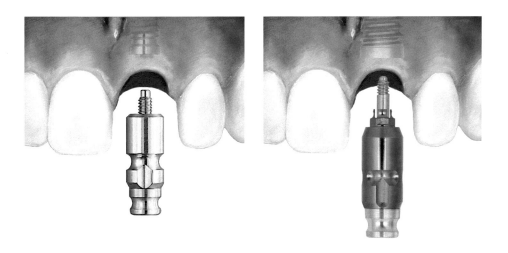

Fig 13-4 The transfer coping is fitted on to the implant.

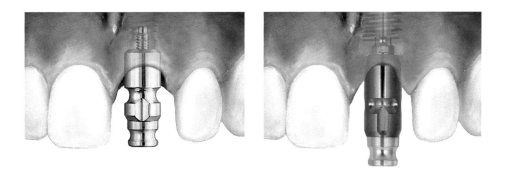

Fig 13-5 The transfer coping attached to the implant.

It is important to ensure that the transfer coping is fully seated on the implant. Usually this cannot be verified directly, and a long cone periapical radiograph (Fig 13-6) should be taken. If a space is evident (*left of each frame*), loosen the screw, slightly rotate the transfer coping until it feels locked into place (*right of each frame*). Retighten the screw by hand and retake the radiograph, if necessary.

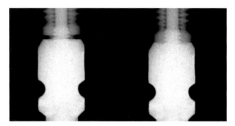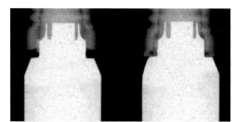

Fig 13-6 Radiograph showing unseated transfer coping (*left of each frame*) and seated coping (*right of each frame*).

The tray can then be filled with impression material. While the tray is being loaded, impression material is carefully syringed around the impression coping and the surrounding soft tissue and teeth (Fig 13-7). This allows the laboratory technician to produce a cast that has an accurate duplication of the soft tissue surrounding the implant. An accurate impression of the tissue will allow the technician to create the final restoration with the correct emergence profile.

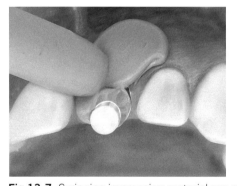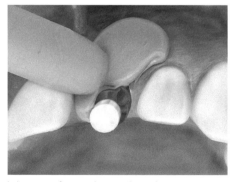

Fig 13-7 Syringing impression material around the transfer coping and teeth.

external	internal

The impression tray is inserted in the mouth over the transfer coping (Fig 13-8). With this technique, the transfer coping does not show through the impression tray.

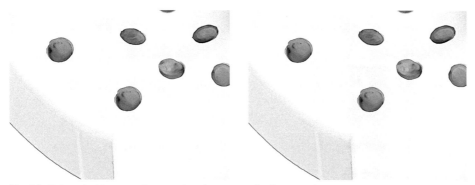

Fig 13-8 Loaded impression tray in place over the impression coping.

Once the impression material has set, it is removed from the mouth. The transfer coping is unscrewed and then placed into the impression to exactly reproduce its original position (Fig 13-9).

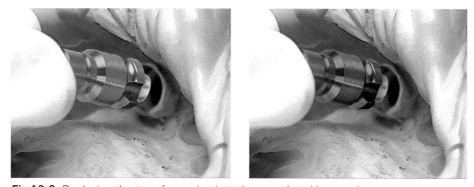

Fig 13-9 Replacing the transfer coping into the completed impression.

external	internal

The impression can then be disinfected prior to sending it to the laboratory technician. Check that the transfer coping is firmly seated in the impression in its correct position (Fig 13-10). If movement of the transfer coping is observed, then its position should be checked or a new impression made.

From this point, the impression is sent to the laboratory and the restoration is completed in the same way as described in the previous chapters in Part 2. At the next visit, the abutment is checked and its fit verified. The restoration is checked for fit, aesthetics, and occlusion, and finally cemented when the operator and patient are satisfied.

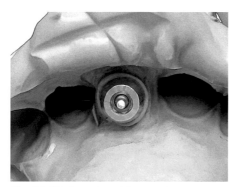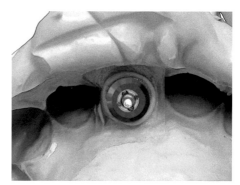

Fig 13-10 Completed impression with transfer coping in position.

Multi-unit Restoration Using a Direct Technique with Preparable Abutments (Metal or Ceramic)

external	internal

Materials and components

- preparable titanium or zirconia posts
- abutment retaining screw
- square driver
- hexagonal driver
- gauze
- periodontal probe or measuring post
- torque indicator
- square or hex tip to go into indicator

- burs (H33L.31.021, 703L.FG, and H158.31.012 H297FG)
- retraction cord
- impression material
- adhesive
- custom tray/stock tray
- immediate restorative material
- bite registration material

Procedure

Remove the provisional healing abutments using a hexagonal screwdriver (Figs 14-1 and 14–2). It is useful to place a square of gauze behind the operating area, as the components are quite small and this prevents possible loss of the abutments if the patient swallows.

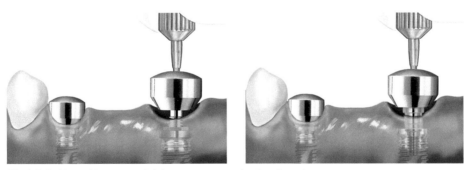

Fig 14-1 Use of hexagonal driver to remove the healing abutments.

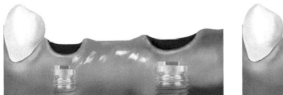
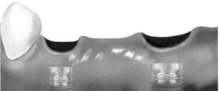

Fig 14-2 Side view of implants with the healing abutments removed.

external	internal

The entire implant platforms should be visible. If there is any soft tissue over the surfaces this should be carefully removed with a plastic- or gold-tipped scaler to avoid damaging the implant surface (Fig 14-3).

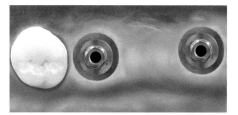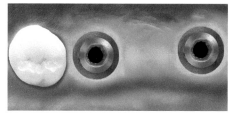

Fig 14-3 Ensure that there is no soft tissue obscuring the implant platform.

To ascertain the height of the collar that is required for the abutments, measure the height of the soft tissue using either a periodontal probe (Fig 14-4) or a tissue measuring post.

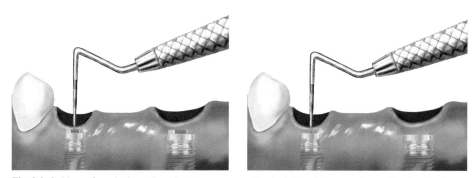

Fig 14-4 Use of periodontal probe to measure the height of tissue above the implant.

Select the abutments that correspond to the platform diameters of the implants and have the appropriate collar height. As a guide, the prepared finish line of the abutments should lie approximately 1 mm below the gingival margin. Place the abutments over the heads of the implants. Slightly rotate the abutments to ensure the hex on the underside of the abutments fully engages the hex of the implants (Fig 14-5). Using the try-in screw and the hexagonal driver, hand tighten the screw to secure the abutments.

| external | internal |

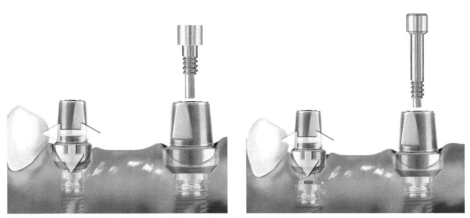

Fig 14-5 Placement of abutment engaging the hex of the implant. The prepared finish line on the abutment should be approximately 1 mm below the soft tissue at the highest point (usually interproximally). Secure the abutment with a try-in screw.

A long cone radiograph is taken to verify that the abutments are fully down onto the head of the implants (Fig 14-6). If a space is evident, loosen the screw, slightly rotate the posts until it feels locked into place. Retighten the screw and retake the radiograph.

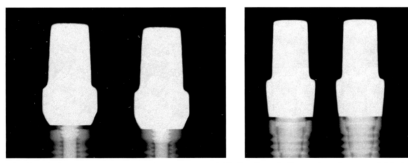

Fig 14-6 Radiographs showing unseated *(left of each frame)* and seated *(right of each frame)* abutments on the implants.

The abutments are then prepared following normal restorative procedures, ensuring that the correct retention and resistance forms are achieved (Fig 14-7). To avoid overpreparation of the abutments, it is recommended that the handpiece is operated at 40,000 rpm. Copious water spray is required to prevent overheating the implant. The abutments are prepared using the following burs:

- H33L.31.021 (Brasseler) for gross cutting in combination with 703L FG (tapered fissure bur)
- H158.31.012 H297FG, which is a carbide finishing bur for final refinement of the abutment.

209

| external | internal |

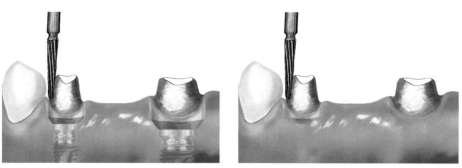

Fig 14-7 Outline preparation of the abutments.

Refinement of the abutment preparations can be completed outside the mouth, using an abutment holder (Fig 14-8). Fine stones and rubber wheels may be used to achieve a smooth finish.

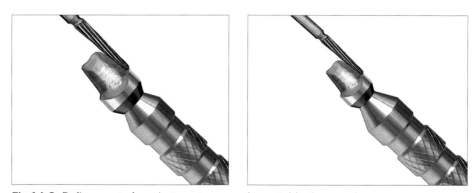

Fig 14-8 Refinement of an abutment preparation outside the mouth.

The abutments are returned to the implants and secured with the appropriate permanent retaining screws (Fig 14-9). A square screw may be used to attach the abutments to the external hex implants, as it can achieve a higher preload. A hexed screw is used to attach the abutments to the internal connection implants.

external	internal

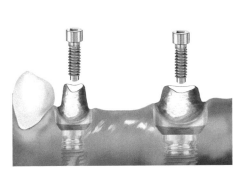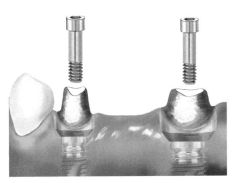

Fig 14-9 Securing the abutment with a permanent screw.

A long cone radiograph is taken to verify that the prepared abutments are fully down on the heads of the implants. Where implants are placed fairly superficially, it may be possible to check the abutment seating visually, or with an instrument, and thereby avoid taking another radiograph. If a space is evident (Fig 14-10, *left of each frame*), loosen the screw, slightly rotate the abutment until it feels locked into place (Fig 14-10, *right of each frame*). Retighten the screw, and retake the radiograph if necessary.

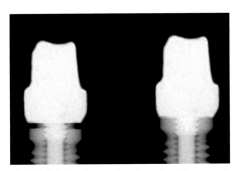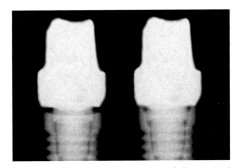

Fig 14-10 Radiographs showing abutments not seated *(left of each frame)* and fully seated *(right of each frame)*.

The square-ended driver tip (external hex implant) or hex-ended driver tip (internal connection implant) is placed in the restorative torque indicator (Fig 14-11). The screw is tightened the correct amount using restorative torque indicator. The restorative torque indicator is rotated clockwise until the triangle on the inner ring and the diamond on the outer ring are coincident; at this point the torque is 35 Ncm (for a square screw) (Fig 14-12a). When the triangle on the inner ring and the triangle on the outer ring are coincident, the torque is 20 Ncm (for a hex screw) (Fig 14-12b).

external   internal

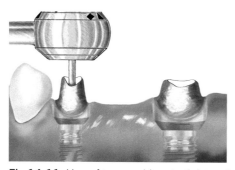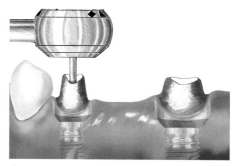

Fig 14-11 Use of torque driver to tighten the abutment screw.

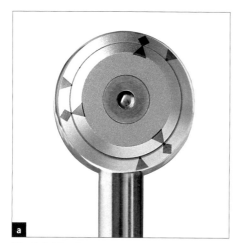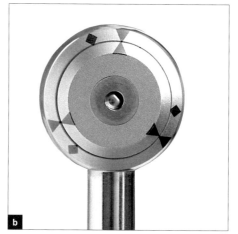

Fig 14-12 Restorative torque indicator showing marks for the application of different torques to screws. The triangle on the inner ring aligned with the diamond on the outer ring gives 35 Ncm torque (a), and aligned with the triangle on the outer ring gives 20 Ncm torque (b).

The access hole is first filled with silicone material or PTFE tape, followed by an intermediate restorative material. This ensures that when the final impression is made, the material will not enter the screw hole and cause distortion of the impression (Fig 14-13).

external	internal

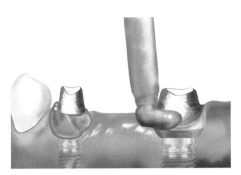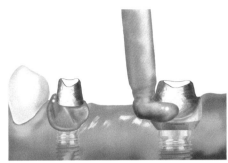

Fig 14-13 Impression being made of prepared abutments.

Retraction cord is placed into the gingival sulcus. This retracts the tissue to enable the operator to see the entire finish line prior to making an impression; it also allows any further minor adjustments to the abutment to be made.

Once retraction of the tissue has been achieved, an impression is made using an impression material of the operator's choice (Fig 14-14). An opposing impression is made together with an interocclusal record and shade prescription for the laboratory technician.

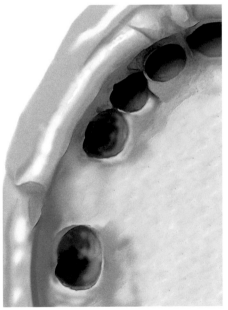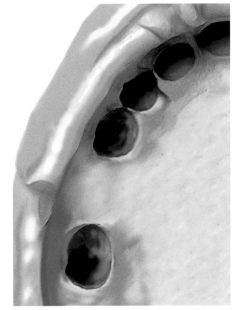

Fig 14-14 Impression of prepared abutments.

external	internal

Provisional restorations may be constructed on each abutment using a preformed crown, relined with a resin material (Fig 14-15). Once this material has set, it can be adjusted, polished, and then cemented to the abutments with a temporary cement.

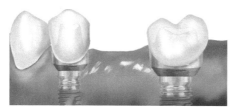 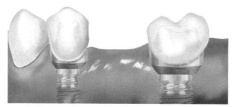

Fig 14-15 Provisional restorations in place on the prepared abutments.

In the laboratory, dies are prepared from the impression to construct the final restoration (Fig 14-16).

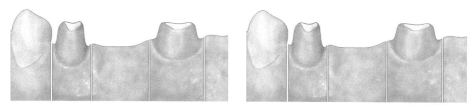

Fig 14-16 Preparing dies for the definitive restoration.

external		internal

The restoration is returned to the clinician (Fig 14-17), ready for insertion.

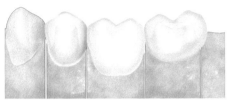 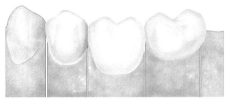

Fig 14-17 Completed restoration on the cast.

The restoration is then tried in the mouth to check shade, contour, and occlusion. It is then cemented over the abutments using either temporary or long-term cement (Fig 14-18). Temporary cement allows for retrievability of the restoration should one of the abutment screws become loose.

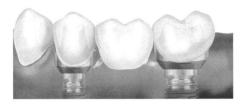 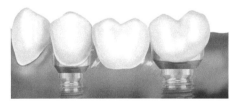

Fig 14-18 Final restoration checked and cemented onto the implant abutments.

Multi-unit Restoration Using an Indirect Technique with Preparable Abutments (Metal or Ceramic)

external		internal	

Materials and components

- hexagonal driver
- square driver
- impression tray
- impression coping with guide pin
- adhesive
- impression material

- restorative torque indicator with square or hexed driver tip
- occlusal registration material
- locking tweezers
- cement material

Procedure

Remove the provisional healing abutments using a hexagonal screwdriver (Figs 15-1 and 15-2). It is useful to place a square of gauze behind the operating area, as the components are quite small and this prevents possible loss of the abutments if the patient swallows.

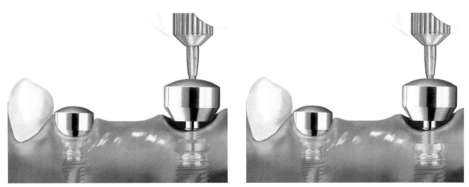

Fig 15-1 Use of hexagonal driver to remove the healing abutments.

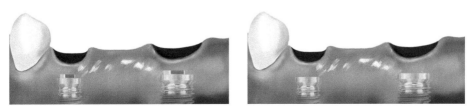

Fig 15-2 Side view of implants with the healing abutments removed.

external	internal

The entire implant platforms should be visible. If there is any soft tissue over the surfaces this should be carefully removed with a plastic- or gold-tipped scaler to avoid damaging the implant surface (Fig 15-13).

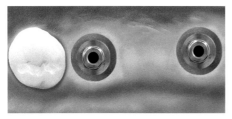 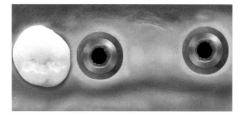

Fig 15-3 Ensure that there is no soft tissue obscuring the implant platform.

Implant impression copings and guide pins are seated onto the fitting surfaces of the implants (Fig 15-4).

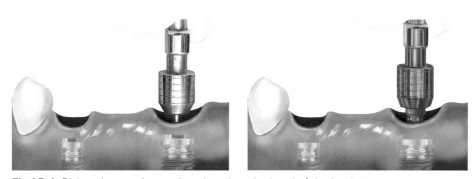

Fig 15-4 Pick-up impression coping placed on the head of the implant.

The impression coping guide pins are then hand tightened and secured using a hexagonal driver (Fig 15-5).

external	internal

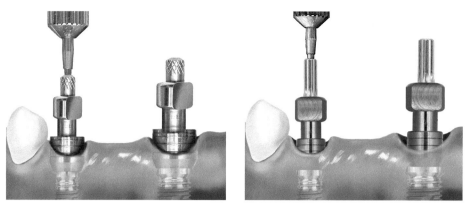

Fig 15-5 Hand tightening of the impression copings with the hexagonal driver.

It is important to ensure that each impression coping assembly is fully seated on the implants. Usually this cannot be verified directly, and a long cone periapical radiograph should be taken. If a space is evident (Fig 15-6, *left of each frame*), loosen the guide pin and slightly rotate the impression coping until it feels locked into place (Fig 15-6, *right of each frame*). Retighten the guide pin and retake the radiograph, if necessary.

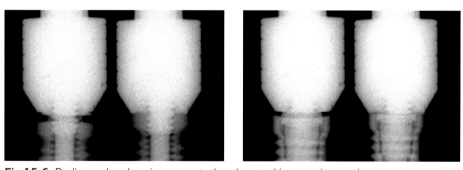

Fig 15-6 Radiographs showing unseated and seated impression copings.

A hole is made in the impression tray and the tray is tried in to ensure that the guide pins protrude through the opening. The guide pin openings may be sealed with pink modeling wax (Fig 15-7). This helps to support the impression material around the impression coping assembly. The tray is then uniformly coated with a thin layer of adhesive, corresponding to the impression material that is going to be used, and allowed to dry.

external	internal

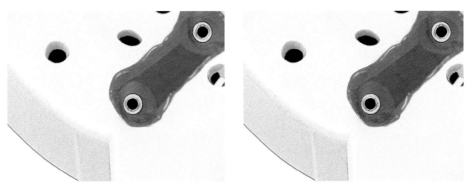

Fig 15-7 Open tray with impression coping guide pins showing through and wax added, if necessary, to prevent the impression material from flowing out.

The tray can then be filled with impression material. While the tray is being loaded, impression material is carefully syringed around the impression copings and the surrounding soft tissue (Fig 15-8). This is essential, as it allows the laboratory technician to produce a cast that has an accurate duplication of the soft tissue surrounding the implant. An accurate impression of the tissue will allow the technician to create a final restoration with the correct emergence profile.

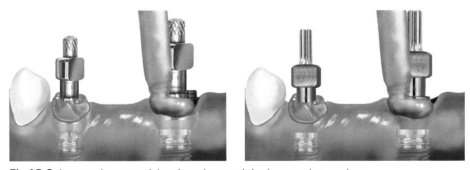

Fig 15-8 Impression material syringed around the impression copings.

The filled tray is then inserted into the mouth, ensuring that the guide pins are visible and protrude through the pink wax on the custom tray (Fig 15-9).

external	internal

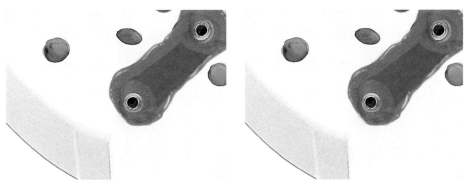

Fig 15-9 Impression coping screw visible through the wax in the "open" tray.

When the material has set, the impression coping pins are unscrewed using a hexagonal driver (Fig 15-10). It is essential that the pins be fully disengaged from the implants before the impression is removed from the mouth.

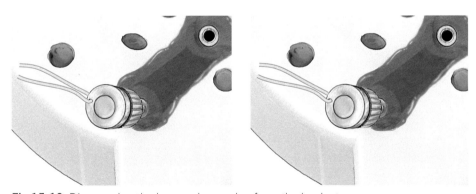

Fig 15-10 Disengaging the impression coping from the implant.

Disengagement of the guide pins is verified by gently lifting the pins with a pair of locking tweezers (Fig 15-11). The pins should move freely without resistance.

external	internal

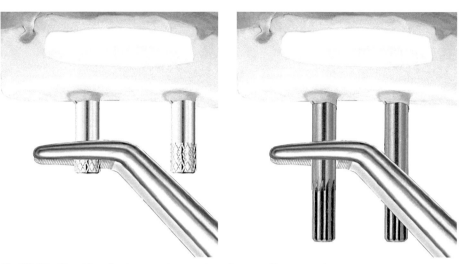

Fig 15-11 Checking the impression coping pins are disengaged.

The impression can then be removed from the mouth (Fig 15-12) and disinfected prior to sending it to the laboratory. It is important to check that the impression copings are firmly embedded in the impression so that no movement of the copings is evident. If the copings move in the impression, the procedure should be repeated.

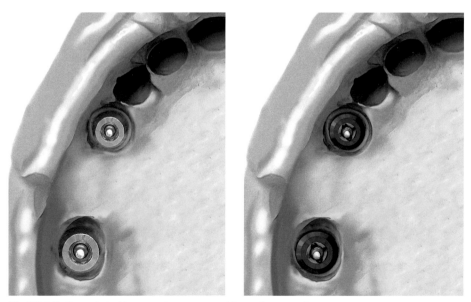

Fig 15-12 Completed impression removed from the mouth.

The provisional healing abutments are replaced and tightened using a hexagonal driver (Fig 15-13). It is essential that the abutments be fully seated down onto the implant to ensure that no soft tissue will proliferate between the abutment and implant. An opposing impression is made together with an interocclusal record and shade prescription for the laboratory technician. If the patient has a provisional restoration, it should be checked and reinserted.

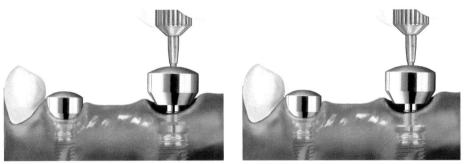

Fig 15-13 Replacing the healing abutment on the implant after removal of the impression.

The laboratory returns the prepared abutments, the locating jig, the try-in screws, the final retaining abutment screws, and the definitive restoration (Fig 15-14).

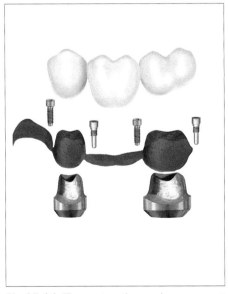 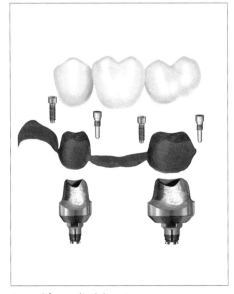

Fig 15-14 The restoration and components returned from the laboratory.

| external | internal |

It is important that the abutments be correctly orientated when finally screwed down on to the head of the implant. This is achieved by the construction of a locating jig (Fig 15-15). The jig is made in the laboratory, using a quick-cure laboratory resin, after the abutments have been prepared by the technician.

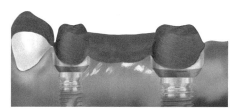 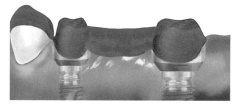

Fig 15-15 Use of locating jig to correctly orientate the abutments on the implants.

The jig should fit accurately over the prepared abutments and should also locate over the adjacent teeth to provide stability. The jig securely holds the abutments in place while the try-in screws are tightened using a hexed driver (Fig 15-16).

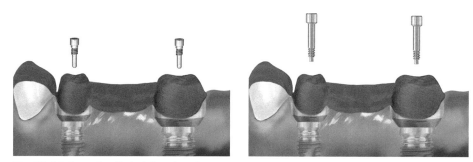

Fig 15-16 Locating jig holding the abutments on the implants to allow try-in screw placement.

A long cone radiograph is taken to verify that the prepared abutments are fully seated on to the head of the implants (Fig 15-17). If a space is evident (*left of each frame*), the master cast is inaccurate and the impression must be retaken (*right of each frame*).

external	internal

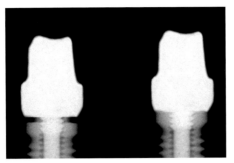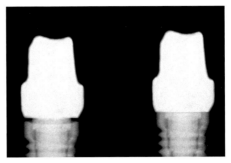

Fig 15-17 Radiographs to verify full seating of the abutments.

Once the seating of the abutments has been verified radiographically, the locating jig is removed, leaving the abutments in position (Fig 15-18).

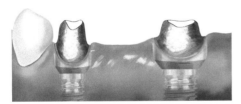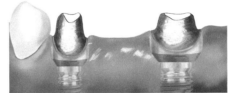

Fig 15-18 Prepared abutments in position.

The final restoration is then tried in the mouth to verify the contour, aesthetics, function, and occlusion (Fig 15-19).

external	internal

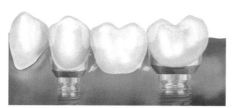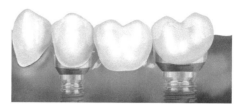

Fig 15-19 Try-in of final restoration.

When the operator is satisfied with the restoration, it is removed and the locating jig repositioned on the abutments. The try-in screws are then removed and replaced with the final abutment retaining screws, which are hand tightened with the appropriate driver (Fig 15-20). For an external hex implant, a square screw may be used, whereas a hexagonal screw is placed on the internal connection implant.

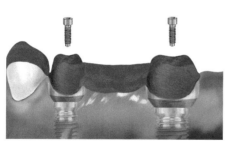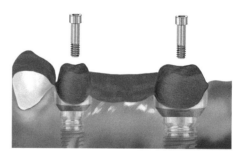

Fig 15-20 Final abutment screws are placed.

external	internal

The square-ended driver tip (external hex implant) or hex-ended driver tip (internal connection implant) is placed in the restorative torque indicator (Fig 15-21). The screw is tightened using the indicator to 35 Ncm (external) or 20 Ncm (internal). The restorative torque indicator is rotated clockwise until the triangle on the inner ring and the diamond on the outer ring are coincident; at this point the torque is 35 Ncm (external hex) (Fig 15-22a). When the triangle on the inner ring and the triangle on the outer ring are coincident, the torque is 20 Ncm (internal connection) (Fig 15-22b).

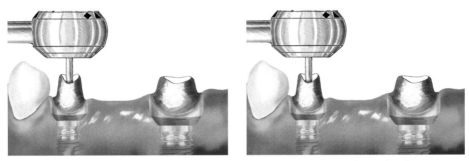

Fig 15-21 Use of torque driver to tighten the abutment screws to the optimal torque.

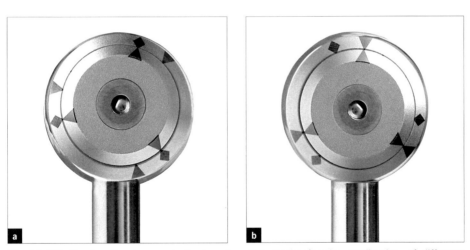

Fig 15-22 Restorative torque indicator showing marks for the application of different torques to the abutment screw. The triangle on the inner ring aligned with the diamond on the outer ring gives 35 Ncm torque (a), and aligned with the triangle on the outer ring gives 20 Ncm torque (b).

external	internal

The screw access holes are filled with either silicone or PTFE material. The restoration is then cemented over the abutments using either temporary or long-term cement (Fig 15-23). Temporary cement makes it easier to retrieve the restoration should one of the abutment screws become loose.

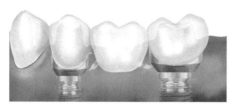 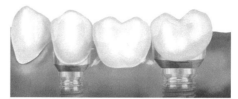

Fig 15-23 Final restoration cemented in place.

Multi-unit Restoration Using UCLA Abutments

external	internal

Materials and components

- square driver
- hexagonal driver
- stock/custom tray
- adhesive impression material

- impression coping and guide pin
- modeling pink wax
- wax knife

Procedure

Remove the provisional healing abutments using a hexagonal screwdriver (Figs 16-1 and 16-2). It is useful to place a square of gauze behind the operating area, as the components are quite small and this prevents possible loss of the abutments if the patient swallows.

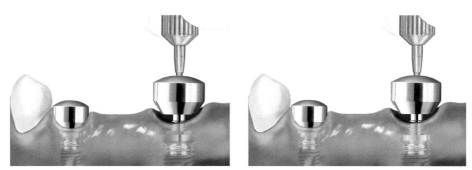

Fig 16-1 Use of hexagonal driver to remove the healing abutments.

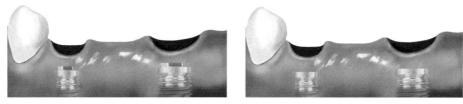

Fig 16-2 Side view of implants with the healing abutments removed.

external	internal

The entire implant platforms should be visible. If there is any soft tissue over the surfaces this should be carefully removed with a plastic- or gold-tipped scaler to avoid damaging the implant surface (Fig 16-3). Implant impression copings and guide pins are placed over the head of the implants (Fig 16-4) and the impression copings are aligned.

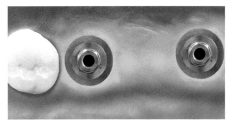 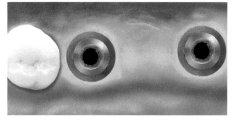

Fig 16-3 Ensure that there is no soft tissue obscuring the implant platform.

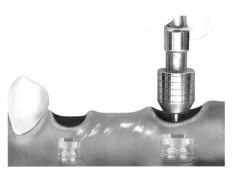 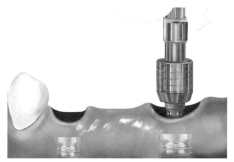

Fig 16-4 Pick-up impression coping placed on the head of the implant.

The impression coping guide pins are then hand tightened and secured using a hexagonal driver (Fig 16-5). It is important to ensure that each impression coping assembly is fully seated on the implant. Usually this cannot be verified directly, and a long cone periapical radiograph should be taken. If a space is evident (Fig 16-6, *left of each frame*), loosen the guide pin and slightly rotate the impression coping until it feels locked into place (Fig. 16-6, *right of each frame*). Retighten the guide pin and retake the radiograph, if necessary.

external	internal

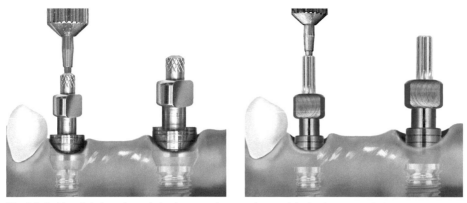

Fig 16-5 Hand tightening of the impression copings with the hexagonal driver.

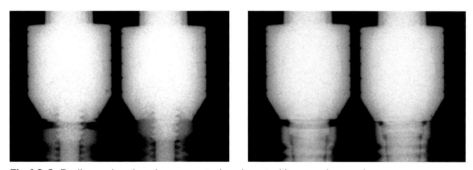

Fig 16-6 Radiographs showing unseated and seated impression copings.

A hole is made in the impression tray and the tray is tried in to ensure that the guide pins protrude through the opening (Fig 16-7). The opening for the guide pins may be sealed with pink modeling wax. This helps to support the impression material around the impression coping assembly. The tray is then uniformly coated with a thin layer of adhesive, corresponding to the impression material that is going to be used, and allowed to dry.

external	internal

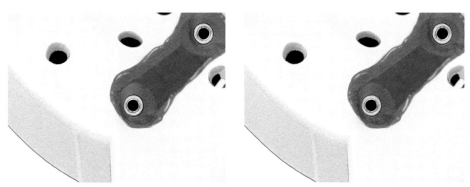

Fig 16-7 Open tray with impression coping guide pins showing through.

The tray can then be filled with impression material. While the tray is being loaded, impression material is carefully syringed around the impression copings and the surrounding soft tissue (Fig 16-8). This is essential, as it allows the laboratory technician to produce a cast that has an accurate duplication of the soft tissue surrounding the implant. An accurate impression of the tissue will allow the technician to create a final restoration with the correct emergence profile.

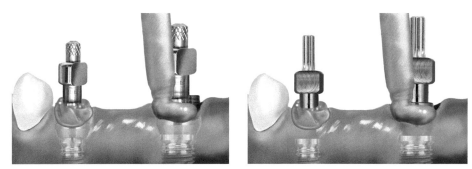

Fig 16-8 Impression material syringed around the impression copings.

The filled tray is then inserted into the mouth, ensuring that the guide pins are visible and protrude through the pink wax on the custom tray (Fig 16-9).

external	internal

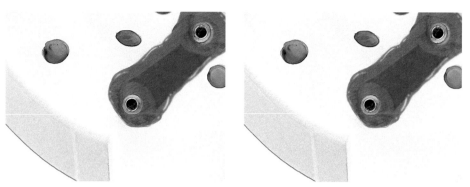

Fig 16-9 Impression coping screw visible through the wax in the open tray.

When the material has set, the impression coping pins are unscrewed using a hexagonal driver (Fig 16-10). It is essential that the pins be fully disengaged from the implants before the impression is removed from the mouth.

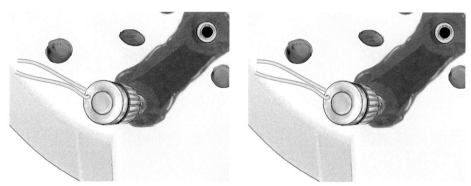

Fig 16-10 Disengaging the impression coping from the implant.

Disengagement of the guide pins is verified by gently lifting the pins with a pair of locking tweezers (Fig 16-11). The pins should move freely without resistance.

| external | internal |

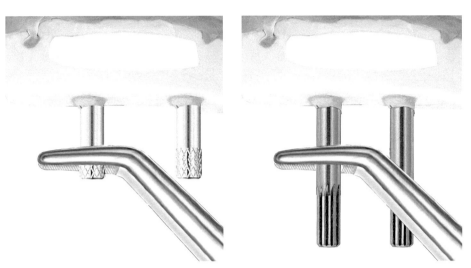

Fig 16-11 Checking the impression coping pins are disengaged.

The impression can then be removed from the mouth (Fig 16-12) and disinfected prior to sending it to the laboratory. It is important to check that the impression copings are firmly embedded in the impression so that no movement of the copings is evident. If the copings move in the impression, the procedure should be repeated.

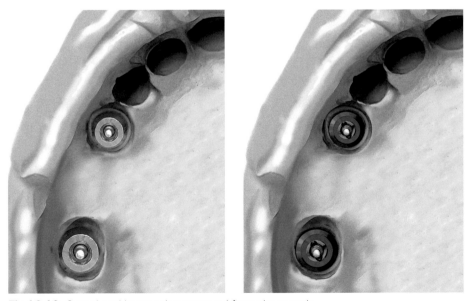

Fig 16-12 Completed impression removed from the mouth.

external	internal

The provisional healing abutments are replaced and tightened using a hexagonal driver (Fig 16-13). It is essential that the abutments be fully seated down onto the implant to ensure that no soft tissue will proliferate between the abutment and implant. An opposing impression is made together with an interocclusal record and shade prescription for the laboratory technician. If the patient has a provisional restoration, it should be checked and reinserted.

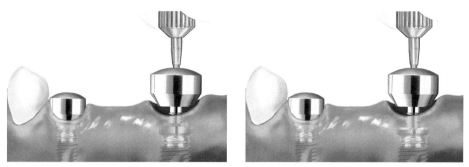

Fig 16-13 Replacing the healing abutment on the implant after removal of the impression.

The laboratory returns the completed UCLA abutments, the locating jig, the try-in screws, the final abutment retaining screws, and the definitive restoration (Fig 16-14).

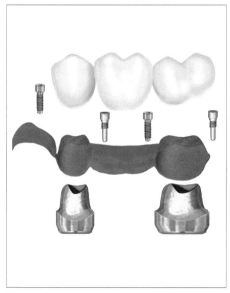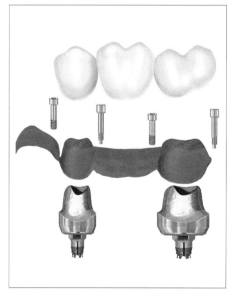

Fig 16-14 Restoration and components ready for try-in

external	internal

It is important that the UCLA abutments be correctly orientated when finally screwed down on to the head of the implant. This is achieved by the construction of a locating jig (Fig 16-15). The jig is made in the laboratory, using a quick-cure laboratory resin, after the abutments have been prepared by the technician.

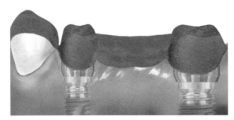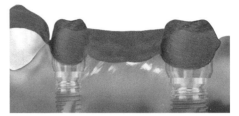

Fig 16-15 Locating jig used to seat the cast UCLA abutments on the implants.

The jig should fit accurately over the UCLA abutments and should also locate over the adjacent teeth to provide stability. The jig securely holds the abutments in place while the try-in screws are tightened using a hexed driver (Fig 16-16).

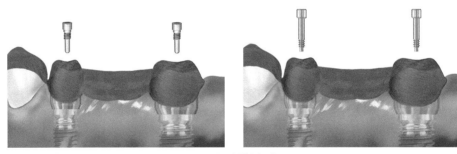

Fig 16-16 Try-in screws used to secure the UCLA abutments.

A long cone radiograph is taken to verify that the UCLA abutment is fully down on to the head of the implant. If a space is evident (Fig 16-17, *left of each frame*), the master cast is inaccurate and, therefore, the impression must be retaken. A fully seated abutment is shown on the *right of each frame*.

| external | internal |

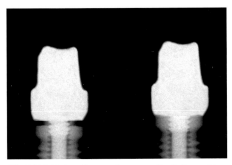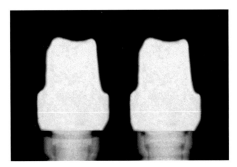

Fig 16-17 Radiograph to verify full seating of the UCLA abutment on the implant.

Once the seating of the abutments has been verified radiographically, the locating jig is removed (Fig 16-18). The definitive restoration is then tried in the mouth to verify the contour, aesthetics, function, and occlusion (Fig 16-19).

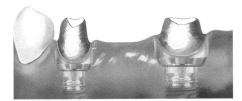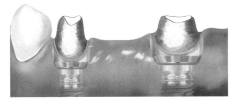

Fig 16-18 Verified UCLA abutments on the implants.

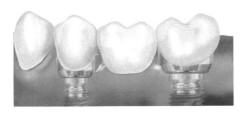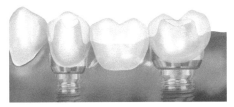

Fig 16-19 Try-in of definitive restoration on the abutments.

external	internal

When the restoration is completed, it is removed and the locating jig is repositioned, if necessary, on the UCLA abutments. The try-in screws are then removed and replaced with the final abutment retaining screws, which are tightened by hand with the driver (Fig 16-20). A square-headed screw may be used on the external hex implant to achieve higher preload, while a hexed screw is used on the internal connection implant.

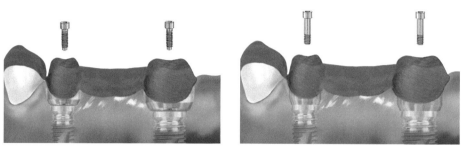

Fig 16-20 Placement of final screws to secure the UCLA abutments.

The driver tip is placed into the restorative torque indicator (Fig 16-21). The square screw (external hex implant) is tightened to 35 Ncm, while the hexed screw (internal connection implant) is tightened to 20 Ncm. The restorative torque indicator is rotated clockwise until the triangle on the inner ring and the diamond on the outer ring are coincident; at this point the torque is 35 Ncm (external hex) (Fig 16-22a). When the triangle on the inner ring and the triangle on the outer ring are coincident, the torque is 20 Ncm (internal connection) (Fig 16-22b).

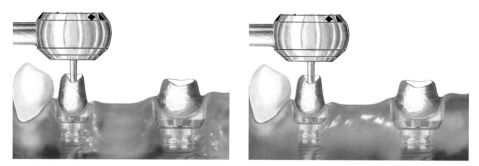

Fig 16-21 Use of torque driver to tighten the abutment screw to the optimal torque.

external | internal

external | internal

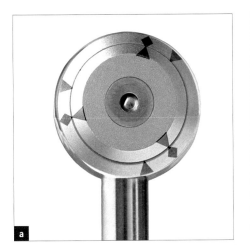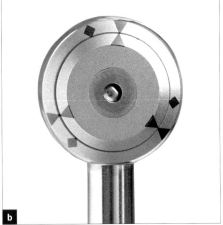

Fig 16-22 Restorative torque indicator showing marks for the application of different torques to the abutment screw. The triangle on the inner ring aligned with the diamond on the outer ring gives 35 Ncm torque (a), and aligned with the triangle on the outer ring gives 20 Ncm torque (b).

The screw access hole in the abutment is sealed with silicone material, wax, or PTFE tape. The crown is then cemented over the abutment using either temporary or long-term cement (Fig 16-23). Temporary cement allows the restoration to be retrieved more easily if the abutment screw becomes loose.

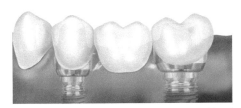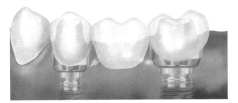

Fig 16-23 Final restoration cemented in place.

Multi-unit Restoration Using Conical Abutments

| external | internal |

Material and components required

- hexagonal driver
- impression tray
- impression material
- periodontal probe or measuring post
- impression coping with guide pin
- restorative torque indicator with conical abutment driver tip

- abutment hand driver
- occlusal registration material
- gauze square
- retaining screw

Procedure

Remove the provisional healing abutments using a hexagonal screwdriver (Figs 17-1 and 17–2). It is useful to place a square of gauze behind the operating area, as the components are quite small and this prevents possible loss of the abutments if the patient swallows.

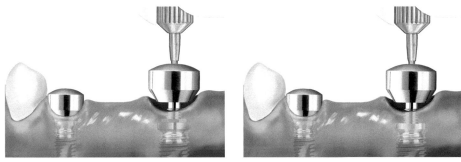

Fig 17-1 Use of hexagonal driver to remove the healing abutments.

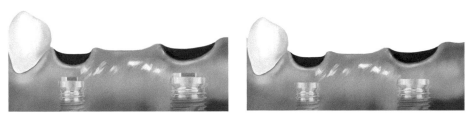

Fig 17-2 Side view of implants with the healing abutments removed.

external	internal

The entire implant platforms should be visible. If there is any soft tissue over the surfaces this should be carefully removed with a plastic- or gold-tipped scaler to avoid damaging the implant surface (Fig 17-13).

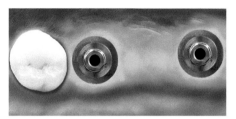 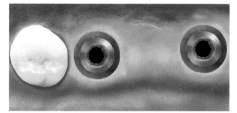

Fig 17-3 Ensure that there is no soft tissue obscuring the implant platform.

To ascertain the height of the collar that is required for the abutments, measure the height of the soft tissue using either a periodontal probe (Fig 17-4) or a tissue measuring post.

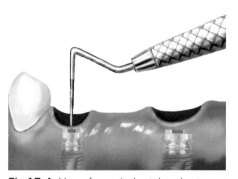 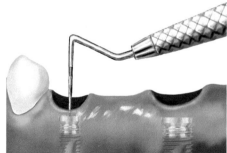

Fig 17-4 Use of a periodontal probe to measure the height of tissue above the implant.

external	internal

The conical abutment is supplied in a sterilizing pouch with an integral disposable driver (Fig 17-5). The abutment is a two-piece unit, consisting of a collar that engages the hexagon of the implant and a screw that secures the abutment to the implant (Fig 17-6).

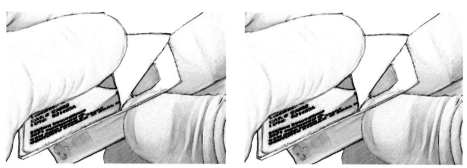

Fig 17-5 Removal of conical abutment with attached plastic driver from pouch.

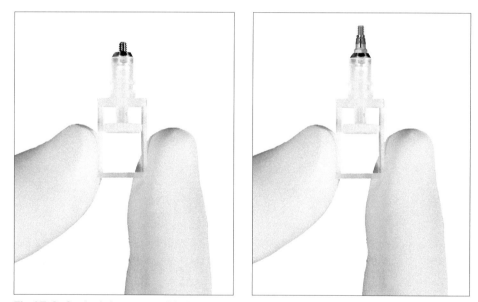

Fig 17-6 Conical abutment with disposable driver.

The collar of the abutment is located over the head of the implant and fully seated to engage the hex (Fig 17-7). It is possible to feel that the abutment seat is fully on the implant.

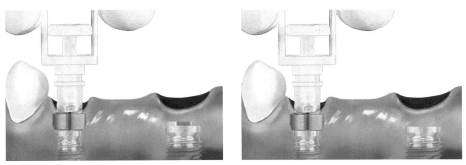

Fig 17-7 Seating the conical abutment on to the head of the implant.

Once the collar is fully seated, the central screw is tightened down manually using the plastic driver (Fig 17-8).

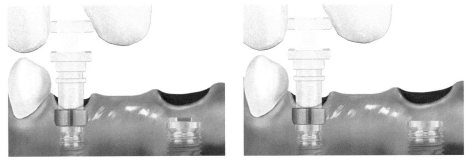

Fig 17-8 Hand-tightening the abutment screw.

The seating of the conical abutment collar on the implant is verified using a long cone radiograph. If the abutment is not seated fully (Fig 17-9, *left of each frame*), then the central abutment screw should be loosened slightly and the abutment rotated until it engages the head of the implant.

external	internal

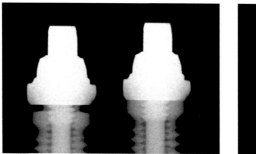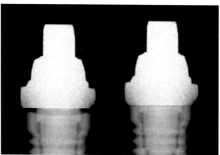

Fig 17-9 Radiograph showing conical abutment not fully seated *(left of each frame)* and completely seated *(right of each frame)*.

The conical abutment is hand tightened using an abutment driver that is designed to fit over the abutment screw (Fig 17-10).

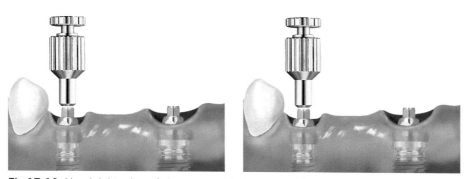

Fig 17-10 Hand tightening of abutment with abutment driver.

The conical abutment driver tip is placed into the restorative torque indicator (Fig 17-11). The screws are tightened using the indicator, which is rotated clockwise until the triangle on the inner ring and the triangle on the outer ring are coincident (Fig 17-12); this gives the required torque of 20 Ncm.

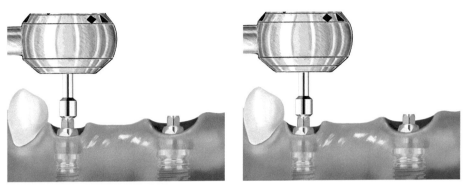

external   internal

Fig 17-11 Use of abutment driver with the restorative torque indicator to tighten the abutment screws.

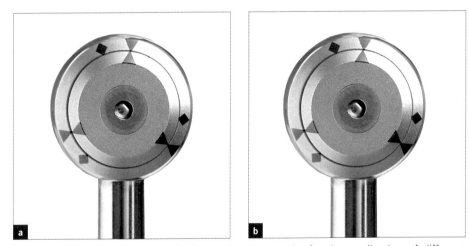

Fig 17-12 Restorative torque indicator showing marks for the application of different torques. The triangle on the inner ring aligned with the diamond on the outer ring gives 35 Ncm torque (a), and aligned with the triangle on the outer ring gives 20 Ncm torque (b).

The impression coping assemblies are placed over the abutments and the guide pins tightened using a hexagonal driver (Fig 17-13). It is important to remember that the impression coping fits over the conical abutment and not directly onto the head of the implant. The coping has no hexagonal configuration internally as the multi-unit restoration does not require an anti-rotational feature.

external | internal

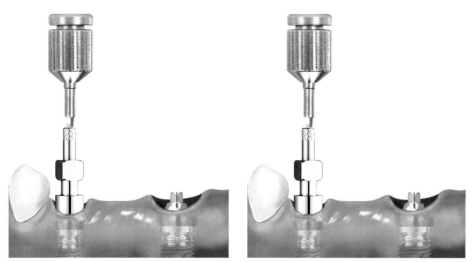

Fig 17-13 Hand tightening of conical abutment impression copings with hex driver.

It is essential to verify that the impression coping assemblies are fully seated on the abutments. Usually this is possible to do directly, but if there is any uncertainty, a long cone periapical radiograph will be required.

Holes are made in the impression tray and the tray is tried in to ensure that the impression coping guide pins protrude through the openings (Fig 17-14). The guide pin openings may be sealed with pink modeling wax. This helps to support the impression material around the impression coping assembly. The tray is then uniformly coated with a thin layer of adhesive, corresponding to the impression material that is going to be used, and allowed to dry.

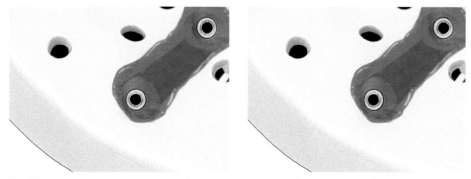

Fig 17-14 Impression tray with holes to accommodate impression coping guide pins.

The tray can then be filled with impression material. While the tray is being loaded, impression material is carefully syringed around the impression copings and the surrounding soft tissue (Fig 17-15). This allows the laboratory technician to produce a cast that has an accurate duplication of the soft tissue surrounding the implant. An accurate impression of the tissue will allow the technician to create the final restoration with the correct emergence profile.

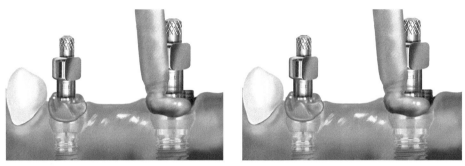

Fig 17-15 Impression material syringed around impression copings and teeth.

The filled tray is then inserted into the mouth, ensuring that the guide pin is visible and protrudes through the pink wax on the custom tray (Fig 17-16).

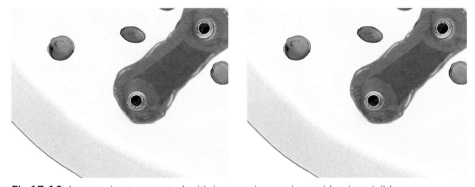

Fig 17-16 Impression tray seated with impression coping guide pins visible.

When the material has set, the guide pins are unscrewed using a hexagonal driver (Fig 17-17). It is essential that the guide pins be fully disengaged from the abutments before the impression is removed from the mouth.

external	internal

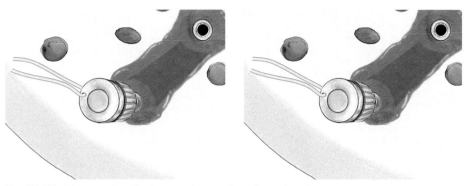

Fig 17-17 Disengaging the impression copings from the abutment.

Check that the guide pins are disengaged from the abutments by gently sliding them away with a locking tweezers (Fig 17-18).

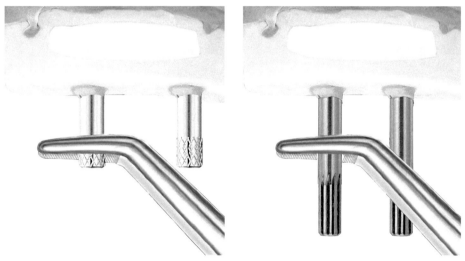

Fig 17-18 Checking the impression coping pins are disengaged.

The impression can then be removed from the mouth (Fig 17-19) and disinfected prior to sending it to the laboratory. Check that the impression copings are firmly embedded in the impression so that no movement of the copings is evident. If the copings move in the impression, the procedure should be repeated.

external	internal

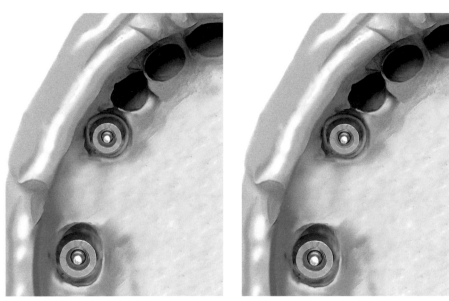

Fig 17-19 Completed impression with copings securely in place.

Temporary healing caps are placed over the conical abutments and tightened using a hexagonal driver (Fig 17-20). An opposing impression is made together with an interocclusal record and shade prescription for the laboratory technician. If the patient has a provisional restoration, it should be checked and reinserted.

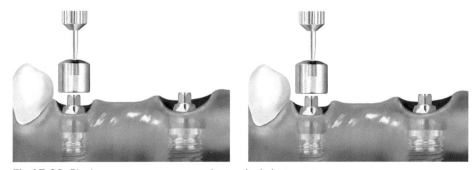

Fig 17-20 Placing temporary caps on the conical abutments.

external	internal

Once the definitive restoration is returned from the laboratory, the temporary caps are removed with the hexagonal driver. The fixed dental prosthesis is tried in to verify fit, contour, occlusion, and aesthetics (Fig 17-21).

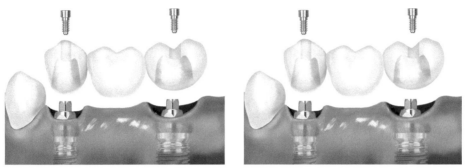

Fig 17-21 Try-in of the restoration using the retaining screws.

A passive fit of the restoration should be verified. When one retaining screw is placed and tightened, the restoration should remain fully seated on the other conical abutment. Both retaining screws are tightened using a hexagonal driver (Fig 17-22). A torque of 10 Ncm is recommended for the retaining screws, which can be achieved by hand tightening. It is essential that a small square of gauze is placed behind the fixed partial denture to ensure that the patient does not accidentally swallow the small retaining screws.

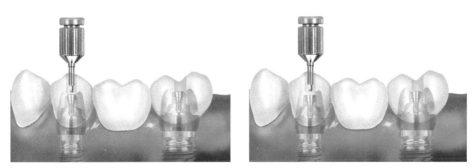

Fig 17-22 Tightening the small retaining screws with a hand driver.

external	internal

The access holes are temporarily filled with a small pledget of cotton wool at the base and covered with an intermediate restorative material. The patient is recalled after 1 week and the intermediate restorative material and cotton wool are removed. The tightness of the retaining screws is verified and the access holes are filled with silicone material or PTFE tape at the base, and at least 2 mm of resin composite on the occlusal surface (Fig 17-23).

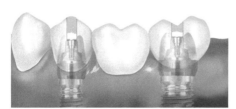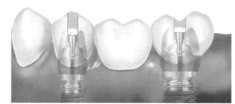

Fig 17-23 Definitive restoration in place with screw access holes sealed.

Multi-unit Restoration Alternative Impression Technique Using Transfer Copings (Closed-tray Technique)

external	internal

An alternative impression technique is available using transfer impression copings that are designed to remain screwed onto the implants or abutments (e.g. conical abutments) when the impression is removed from the mouth. In this case, access holes for the transfer copings are not required in the impression tray. The transfer coping consists of a central screw that secures an outer cylinder to the implant or abutment. The technique may be used for single- or multi-unit restorations.

The advantages of the transfer coping are that it can be used where there is limited space for a driver and trimming of the impression tray is not required, hence simplifying the procedure. The disadvantage of this technique is that the transfer copings must be repositioned in the impression after it is removed from the mouth. It is sometimes difficult to correctly place the transfer copings in the impression, which will lead to an inaccurate master cast.

The provisional healing abutments are removed using a hexagonal screwdriver (Figs 18-1 and 18–2). It is useful to place a square of gauze behind the operating area, as the components are quite small and this prevents possible loss of the abutments if the patient swallows.

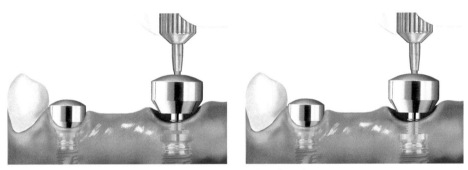

Fig 18-1 Use of hexagonal driver to remove the healing abutments.

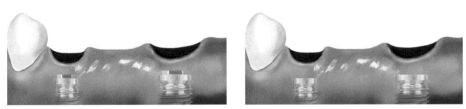

Fig 18-2 Side view of implants with the healing abutments removed.

261

| external | internal |

The entire implant platforms should be visible. Any soft tissue over the surfaces should be carefully removed with a plastic- or gold-tipped scaler to avoid damaging the implant surface (Fig 18-3).

Transfer copings are placed on the implants (Fig 18-4), taking care that the copings align with the external hex or internal connection of the implants.

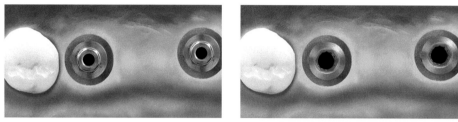

Fig 18-3 Ensure that there is no soft tissue obscuring the implant platform.

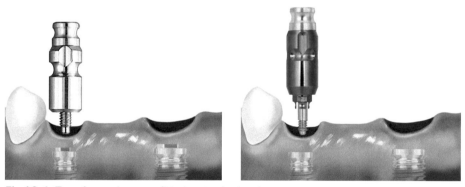

Fig 18-4 Transfer copings are fitted on to the implants.

The transfer copings are finger tightened and checked for stability on the implants (Fig 18-5). It is important to ensure that each transfer coping is fully seated on the implant. Usually this cannot be verified directly, and a long cone periapical radiograph should be taken. If a space is evident (Fig 18-6, *left of each frame*), loosen the screw and slightly rotate the transfer coping until it feels locked into place (Fig 18-6, *right of each frame*). Retighten the screw by hand and retake the radiograph if necessary.

external	internal

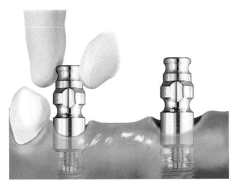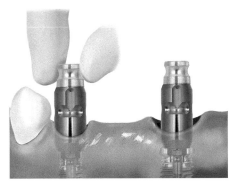

Fig 18-5 Transfer copings attached to the implants.

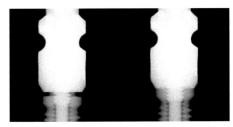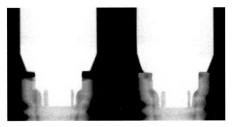

Fig 18-6 Radiograph showing unseated transfer coping *(left of each frame)* and seated coping *(right of each frame)*.

The tray can then be filled with impression material. While the tray is being loaded, impression material is carefully syringed around the impression copings and the surrounding soft tissue (Fig 18-7).

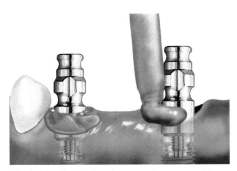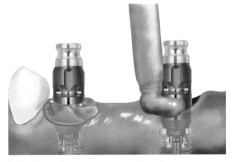

Fig 18-7 Syringing impression material around the transfer copings and teeth.

external	internal

This allows the laboratory technician to produce a cast that has an accurate duplication of the soft tissue surrounding the implant. An accurate impression of the tissue will allow the technician to create the final restoration with the correct emergence profile.

The impression tray is inserted in the mouth over the transfer copings. With this technique, the transfer copings do not show through the impression tray (Fig 18-8).

Once the impression material has set, it is removed from the mouth. The transfer copings are unscrewed and then placed into the impression to exactly reproduce their original positions (Figs 18-9 and 18–10). The impression can then be disinfected prior to sending it to the laboratory. Check that the transfer copings are firmly seated in the impression in their correct position. If movement of the transfer copings is observed, then their position should be checked or a new impression made.

From this point, the impression is sent to the laboratory and the restoration is completed in the same way as before. At the next visit, the abutments are checked and their fit verified. The restoration is checked for fit, aesthetics, and occlusion, and finally cemented when the operator and patient are satisfied.

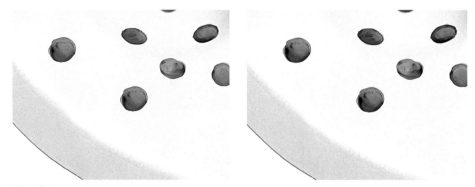

Fig 18-8 Loaded impression tray in place over the impression copings.

| external | internal |

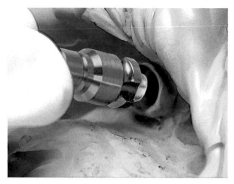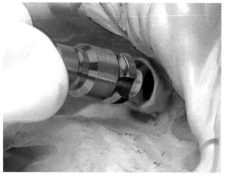

Fig 18-9 Replacing the transfer copings into the completed impression.

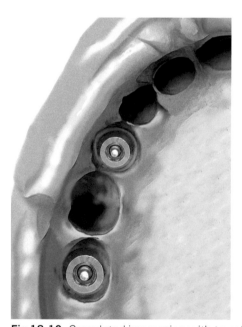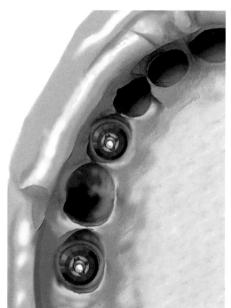

Fig 18-10 Completed impression with transfer copings in position.

Troubleshooting

There are many different complications that may occur in patients with dental implants. It is beyond the scope of this book to catalogue all of the possible problems. The more common clinical complications have been highlighted in this chapter.

Screw loosening

There are two main reasons why screw loosening occurs:
- the incorrect torque is applied to the screw
- there is a mismatch between the diameter of the implant and the width of the crown the final prosthesis replaces.

Incorrect torque

In order to create a stable implant–abutment interface, it is necessary to place the correct preload on to the screw. This involves stretching the material of the screw to 80% of its elastic limit. This allows the screw to return to its original length as the torque is released, hence clamping the two components together. If the screw is tightened by hand, an adequate preload cannot be achieved, which results in the screw not being stretched to its full potential. This will lead to repeated screw loosening. However, if the screw is overtightened and exceeds the elastic limit, it will become plastic and not return to its original length, hence placing no tension into the system. This will lead to loosening and may cause eventual fracture. The design of the screw head impacts on the ability to apply the preload. Slotted screws do not permit an adequate preload to be applied. Square and hexagonal screws allow the preload to be transmitted through the screw, and either can be used.

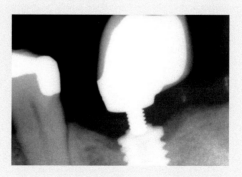

Fig 19-1 Radiograph showing abutment screw loosened with abutment still attached to the crown.

Screw loosening may also occur where the abutment underlying the crown becomes loose, but the crown remains cemented (Fig 19-1). This is sometimes a difficult problem as the crown may not become detached from the abutment easily. If the crown will not separate, it may be possible to cut a hole in the crown to expose the screw access hole underneath. This may be difficult as the access hole may not be in the center of the abutment and so can be difficult to locate. Extensive cutting of the crown may damage the underlying abutment and lead to eventual replacement of the whole assembly. Another method is to cut through the interproximal contacts and create enough space to unscrew the whole assembly. The abutment can then be relocated onto the implant and the screw torqued down. An impression can then be made using conventional crown and fixed partial denture techniques to construct a new restoration.

Solution

Always use a torque driver to tighten screws. This will lead to the correct torque being applied, which will eliminate screw loosening. Always follow the manufacturer's recommendations as to the amount of torque that should be applied. Replace abutment screws that have loosened repeatedly or are damaged.

Mismatch between the diameter of the tooth that is being replaced and the implant

There is always a small mismatch in fit between the top of the implant and the undersurface of the abutment because of the tolerance created by the manufacturers. During function, forces are applied that cause a small amount of movement between the component parts. This is termed micromovement. If the forces that are applied fall outside the diameter of the implant, the movement between the component parts is magnified and the screw is more likely to become loose (Fig 19-2).

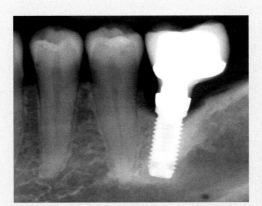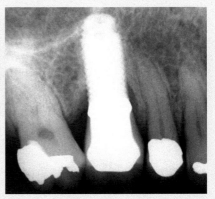

Fig 19-2 A mismatch between the diameter of the implant and the restoration is more likely to cause micromovement at the implant–abutment interface. This can be reduced by selecting an implant that matches the diameter of the tooth being replaced, as closely as possible.

Solution

Always plan the treatment carefully to ensure that the diameter of the implant matches the diameter of the tooth that is being replaced as closely as possible, hence reducing the amount of micro-movement that occurs between the component parts. For multi-unit restorations, choose the correct number of implants to allow even distribution of the forces. It is advisable to use components from the same manufacturer in order to ensure the best fit and stability.

Porcelain or acrylic resin fracture of the superstructure

A fracture in the superstructure is normally caused by failure to design the occlusion correctly, or if the interface between the material and the underlying metal framework is placed under stress. The latter usually happens if the framework is not rigid enough to support the facing material, leading to flexure of the material under occlusal loading. Bruxism parafunctional habits or extensive cantilevering can increase the risk of fractures.

Acrylic resin is slightly more forgiving than porcelain, but if it is too thin it will fracture when loaded. With a screw-retained restoration, the alignment of the retaining screw access hole should ideally be in the central fossa of the restoration to allow an adequate thickness of porcelain or acrylic resin to be applied. Failure to do this will result in inadequate bulk of facing material, leading to possible fracture.

Solution

Check the occlusion in lateral excursions to ensure there are no interferences. If the crown needs to be removed, it is possible either to unscrew the component if it is a screw-retained prosthesis, or to ease it off if it is a cement-retained prosthesis. By cementing the crown with a temporary cement, the removal of the crown can be carried out simply with either Richwill crown removers or rubber-tipped forceps. It must be ensured that the framework is correctly designed, so that it is neither too thin nor too thick. Damage to the prosthesis usually requires complete replacement; hence, careful design is essential to avoid unwanted complications.

Tilted teeth

Tilted teeth may cause poor embrasure and contact areas to be created once the final restoration is constructed. Poor contact areas will lead to food packing, creating gingival inflammation and exaggerated black triangle areas.

Solution

Minor orthodontic uprighting procedures will allow implants to be placed parallel to the long axis of the teeth adjacent to the edentulous space. This allows a restoration to be constructed with the correct contours, contact points, and embrasure spaces, thus promoting gingival health.

Screw fracture

Screw fracture occurs as a result of overloading of the implant by occlusal forces. In this situation, the abutment screws become loose and eventually fracture. Incorrect preload may also create ultimate fracture of the screw. Overtightening of the screw may eventually cause fracture. Excessive cantilever design will also cause occlusal overload and may eventually lead to fracture.

Solution

Screw fracture is very difficult to deal with. It may be possible to remove the screw with specialist equipment. Extreme care must be taken to avoid damaging the internal thread of the implant, which would render the implant unusable for restoration. In the worst case, the implant will need to be removed surgically, the site left to heal, and a new implant placed and then restored once the implant has integrated with the surrounding bone. Fracture of the screw may be related to the design of the superstructure, and careful planning at the design stage should minimize this problem. Avoiding excessive cantilevers and controlling the forces applied to the prosthesis will reduce the problem. If the screw cannot be removed, it may be necessary to drill out the screw in order to salvage the implant. A cemented post and abutment can be constructed from an impression of the internal surface of the implant, and a new superstructure constructed.

Speech

Speech problems may occur as a result of restoration positioning in the buccolingual and labiopalatal planes. Construction of a "hybrid" restoration with spaces between the superstructure and the underlying tissue can cause the escape of air and saliva. This may affect phonetics and speech. Abnormal contouring of the palatal surfaces of the teeth as a result of poor implant alignment may cause an alteration in speech patterns.

Solution

If there has been a lot of tissue loss, it may be possible for the surgeon to carry out graft procedures to eliminate the space. However, great care must be taken to teach the patient hygiene maintenance as cleaning will become more difficult. Redesigning the prosthesis by closing spaces will improve the situation but, again, hygiene must be excellent to maintain gingival health. Keeping the palatal aspect as close as possible to the original contours of the natural teeth will minimize speech difficulties.

Aesthetics

Aesthetic problems are more common in the maxilla. One of the biggest challenges is attempting to place the restored teeth in the position where the natural teeth had previously been. The best results are achieved when the prosthetic teeth are placed in the natural tooth position. Tissue loss can create extra-long teeth, which are unaesthetic. The lost tissue can be recreated using acrylic resin or porcelain. It is essential that the restorations are contoured to allow cleaning around the abutments to maintain the gingival health.

The maintenance of the interdental papilla is essential in creating an aesthetic restoration. Failure to maintain the papilla results in the classic black triangle.

Solution

At the time of implant placement, the head of the implant can be placed slightly deeper than the cementoenamel junction of the adjacent teeth. This will ensure that the interdental tissues will be adequately supported by the relevant healing abutment or provisional restoration prior to the final restoration being placed. Soft tissue can be recontoured at second-stage surgery or after. The construction of a provisional restoration with a contact area more apical than the normal position will support the residual interdental embrasure tissue. This encourages the interdental papilla to mature and potentially creep into the triangular space.

Maintenance after treatment

Following the completion of treatment, maintenance includes regular monitoring, which is similar to that required for a conventional crown and fixed partial denture. Routine radiographic analysis should be carried out to assess bone levels around the implants. Radiographs can both detect loss of crestal bone and verify bone–implant contact along the length of the implant.

Removal of the superstructure to assess the integrity of the implants was thought to be essential in the overall maintenance of the implant–prosthesis complex. However, few practitioners now consider this to be necessary.

Periodontal probing indicates the height of crestal bone–implant contact and the connective tissue attachment. Increased probing depths may indicate progressive bone loss or gingival hyperplasia owing to poor oral hygiene measures. In the case of overdentures, micromovement may cause hyperplasia, particularly when a bar is used as a substructure to support the complete denture.

Plaque control

Poor plaque control can lead to gingival inflammation and, in severe cases, may lead to infection around the implant. Looseness of the abutment can also lead to gingival inflammation and swelling.

Mechanical plaque removal is essential in maintaining soft tissue health around implants. The creation of correctly designed restorations will ensure that cleaning is simple and effective. Patients must be shown how to clean around implants mechanically using traditional techniques. These include traditional toothbrushes, electric brushes, interdental brushes, and floss.

Hardened deposits may develop around implant-borne restorations, and these will require professional cleaning. Specialized scalers with plastic tips or titanium nitride-coated tips can be used. Normal scalers should be avoided as they may scratch the abutment, leading to increased plaque retention.

Chlorhexidine digluconate 0.2% may be used for plaque control. This should only be used for short periods of time, since it may cause extrinsic staining of both soft and hard tissues. It is particularly useful after surgery where the patient may find cleaning difficult.

References

Albrektsson T, Brånemark P-I, Hansson HA, Lindstrom J. Osseointegrated titanium implants: requirements for ensuring a long-lasting, direct bone-to-implant anchorage in man. Acta Orthop Scand 1981;52(2):155–170.

Albrektsson T, Zarb G, Worthington P, Eriksson AR. The long-term efficacy of currently used dental implants: a review and proposed criteria of success. Int J Oral Maxillofac Implants 1986;1(1):11–25.

Astrand P, Engquist B, Dahlgren S, Engquist E, Feldmann H, Grondahl K. Astra Tech and Brånemark System implants: a prospective 5-year comparative study: results after one year. Clin Implant Dent Relat Res 1999;1(1):17–26.

Berglundh T, Persson L, Klinge B. A systematic review of the incidence of biological and technical complications in implant dentistry reported in prospective longitudinal studies of at least 5 years. J Clin Periodontol 2002;29(Suppl 3):197–212; discussion 232–233.

Brånemark P-I, Svensson B, van Steenberghe D. Ten-year survival rates of fixed prostheses on four or six implants ad modum Brånemark in full edentulism. Clin Oral Implants Res 1995;6(4):227–231.

Bryant SR, MacDonald-Jankowski D, Kim K. Does the type of implant prosthesis affect outcomes for the completely edentulous arch? Int J Oral Maxillofac Implants 2007;22(Suppl):117–139.

Buser D, Dula K, Hess D, Hirt HP, Belser UC. Localized ridge augmentation with autografts and barrier membranes. Periodontol 2000 1999;19:151–163.

Choquet V, Hermans M, Adriaenssens P, Daelemans P, Tarnow DP, Malevez C. Clinical and radiographic evaluation of the papilla level adjacent to single-tooth dental implants: a retrospective study in the maxillary anterior region. J Periodontol 2001;72(10):1364–1371.

Dreiseidler T, Mischkowski RA, Neugebauer J, Ritter L, Zoller JE. Comparison of cone-beam imaging with orthopantomography and computerized tomography for assessment in presurgical implant dentistry. Int J Oral Maxillofac Implants 2009;24(2):216–225.

Ericsson I, Randow K, Nilner K, Peterson A. Early functional loading of Brånemark dental implants: 5-year clinical follow-up study. Clin Implant Dent Relat Res 2(2):2000;70–77.

Esposito M, Grusovin MG, Achille H, Coulthard P, Worthington HV. Interventions for replacing missing teeth: different times for loading dental implants. Cochrane Database Syst Rev 2009;(1):CD003878.

Esposito M, Grusovin MG, Chew YS, Coulthard P, Worthington HV. Interventions for replacing missing teeth: 1- versus 2-stage implant placement. Cochrane Database Syst Rev 2009;(3): CD006698.

Esposito M, Grusovin MG, Coulthard P, Worthington HV. The efficacy of various bone augmentation procedures for dental implants: a Cochrane systematic review of randomized controlled clinical trials. Int J Oral Maxillofac Implants 2006;21(5):696–710.

Esposito M, Murray-Curtis L, Grusovin MG, Coulthard P, Worthington HV. Interventions for replacing missing teeth: different types of dental implants. Cochrane Database Syst Rev 2007;(4):CD003815.

Goodacre CJ, Bernal G, Rungcharassaeng K, Kan JY. Clinical complications in fixed prosthodontics. J Prosthet Dent 2003;90(1): 31–41.

Goodacre CJ, Bernal G, Rungcharassaeng K, Kan JY. Clinical complications with implants and implant prostheses. J Prosthet Dent 2003;90(2):121–132.

Gotfredsen K, Berglundh T, Lindhe J. Bone reactions adjacent to titanium implants with different surface characteristics subjected to static load: a study in the dog (II). Clin Oral Implants Res 2001;12(3):196–201.

Gotfredsen K, Karlsson U. A prospective 5-year study of fixed partial prostheses supported by implants with machined and TiO_2-blasted surface. J Prosthodont 2001;10(1):2–7.

Harris D, Buser D, Dula K, Gröndahl K, Harris D, Jacobs R et al. EAO guidelines for the use of diagnostic imaging in implant dentistry. Clin Oral Implants Res 2002;13:566–570.

Lazzara R, Siddiqui AA, Binon P, Feldman SA, Weiner R, Phillips R, et al. Retrospective multicenter analysis of 3i endosseous dental implants placed over a five-year period. Clin Oral Implants Res 1996;7(1):73–83.

Lekholm U, Zarb GA. Patient selection and preparation. In: Brånemark P-I, Zarb GA, Albrektsson T. Tissue-integrated Prostheses: Osseointegration in Clinical Dentistry. Chicago, IL: Quintessence, 1985:199–209.

Moberg LE, Kondell PA, Sagulin GB, Bolin A, Heimdahl A, Gynther GW. Brånemark System and ITI Dental Implant System for treatment of mandibular edentulism: a comparative randomized study: 3-year follow-up. Clin Oral Implants Res 2001;12(5):450–461.

Pjetursson BE, Tan K, Lang NP, Bragger U, Egger M, Zwahlen M. A systematic review of the survival and complication rates of fixed partial dentures (FPDs) after an observation period of at least 5 years. Clin Oral Implants Res 2004;15(6):625–642.

Tarnow DP, Magner AW, Fletcher P. The effect of the distance from the contact point to the crest of bone on the presence or absence of the interproximal dental papilla. J Periodontol 1992;63(12):995–996.

Torabinejad M, Anderson P, Bader J, Brown LJ, Chen LH, Goodacre CJ, et al. Outcomes of root canal treatment and restoration, implant-supported single crowns, fixed partial dentures, and extraction without replacement: a systematic review. J Prosthet Dent 2007;98(4):285–311.

Zarb GA, Schmitt A. The longitudinal clinical effectiveness of osseointegrated dental implants: the Toronto study. Part I: Surgical results. J Prosthet Dent 1990;63(4):451–457.

Zarb GA, Schmitt A. The longitudinal clinical effectiveness of osseointegrated dental implants: the Toronto Study. Part II: The prosthetic results. J Prosthet Dent 1990;64(1):53–61.

Zarb GA, Schmitt A. The longitudinal clinical effectiveness of osseointegrated dental implants: the Toronto study. Part III: Problems and complications encountered. J Prosthet Dent 1990;64(2):185–194.

Further reading

Albrektsson T, Wennerberg A. Oral implant surfaces. Part 1: Review focusing on topographic and chemical properties of different surfaces and in vivo responses to them. Int J Prosthodont 2004;17(5):536–543.

Albrektsson T, Wennerberg A. Oral implant surfaces. Part 2: Review focusing on clinical knowledge of different surfaces. Int J Prosthodont 2004;17(5):544–564.

Albrektsson T, Zarb GA. Current interpretations of the osseointegrated response: clinical significance. Int J Prosthodont 1993;6(2):95–105.

Albrektsson T, Johansson C, Sennerby L. Biological aspects of implant dentistry: osseointegration. Periodontol 2000 1994;4:58–73.

Alsaadi G, Quirynen M, Komarek A, van Steenberghe D. Impact of local and systemic factors on the incidence of oral implant failures, up to abutment connection. J Clin Periodontol 2007; 34(7):610–617.

Bakke M, Holm B, Gotfredsen K. Masticatory function and patient satisfaction with implant-supported mandibular overdentures: a prospective 5-year study. Int J Prosthodont 2002; 15(6):575–581.

Barone A, Covani U, Cornelini R, Gherlone E. Radiographic bone density around immediately loaded oral implants. Clin Oral Implants Res 2003;14(5):610–615.

Boyan BD, Batzer R, Kieswetter K, Liu Y, Cochran DL, Szmuckler-Moncler S, et al. Titanium surface roughness alters responsiveness of MG63 osteoblast-like cells to 1 alpha, 25-(OH)$_2$D$_3$. J Biomed Mater Res 1998;39(1):77–85.

Broggini N, McManus LM, Hermann JS, Medina RU, Oates TW, Schenk RK, et al. Persistent acute inflammation at the implant–abutment interface. J Dent Res 2003;82(3):232–237.

Brunski JB, Moccia AF, Jr, Pollack SR, Korostoff E, Trachtenberg DI. The influence of functional use of endosseous dental implants on the tissue–implant interface. I: Histological aspects. J Dent Res 1979;58(10):1953–1969.

Brunski JB, Moccia AF, Jr, Pollack SR, Korostoff E, Trachtenberg DI. The influence of functional use of endosseous dental implants on the tissue–implant interface. II: Clinical aspects. J Dent Res 1979;58(10):1970–1980.

Buser D, Martin W, Belser UC. Optimizing esthetics for implant restorations in the anterior maxilla: anatomic and surgical considerations. Int J Oral Maxillofac Implants 2004;19(Suppl):43–61.

Buser D, Mericske-Stern R, Dula K, Lang NP. Clinical experience with one-stage, non-submerged dental implants. Adv Dent Res 1999;13:153–161.

Buser D, Nydegger T, Oxland T, Cochran DL, Schenk RK, Hirt HP, et al. Interface shear strength of titanium implants with a sandblasted and acid-etched surface: a biomechanical study in the maxilla of miniature pigs. J Biomed Mater Res 1999;45(2):75–83.

Cochran DL, Hermann JS, Schenk RK, Higginbottom FL, Buser D. Biologic width around titanium implants: a histometric analysis of the implanto-gingival junction around unloaded and loaded nonsubmerged implants in the canine mandible. J Periodontol 1997;68(2):186–198.

Collaert B, De Bruyn H. Early loading of four or five Astra Tech fixtures with a fixed cross-arch restoration in the mandible. Clin Implant Dent Relat Res 2002;4(3):133–135.

Covani U, Cornelini R, Barone A. Bucco-lingual bone remodeling around implants placed into immediate extraction sockets: a case series. J Periodontol 2003;74(2):268–273.

Davarpanah M, Martinez H, Tecucianu JF, Celletti R, Lazzara R. Small-diameter implants: indications and contraindications. J Esthet Dent 2000;12(4):186–194.

Davis DM, Zarb GA, Chao YL. Studies on frameworks for osseointegrated prostheses. Part 1: The effect of varying the number of supporting abutments. Int J Oral Maxillofac Implants 1988;3(3): 197–201.

De Bruyn H, Collaert B. The effect of smoking on early implant failure. Clin Oral Implants Res 1994;5(4):260–264.

De Bruyn H, Collaert B. Early loading of machined-surface Brånemark implants in completely edentulous mandibles: healed bone versus fresh extraction sites. Clin Implant Dent Relat Res 2002;4(3):136–142.

Ericsson I, Johansson CB, Bystedt H, Norton MR. A histomorphometric evaluation of bone-to-implant contact on machine-prepared and roughened titanium dental implants: a pilot study in the dog. Clin Oral Implants Res 1994;5(4):202–206.

Esposito M, Koukoulopoulou A, Coulthard P, Worthington HV. Interventions for replacing missing teeth: dental implants in fresh extraction sockets (immediate, immediate-delayed and delayed implants). Cochrane Database Syst Rev 2006;(4):CD005968.

Fiorellini JP, Buser D, Paquette DW, Williams RC, Haghighi D, Weber HP. A radiographic evaluation of bone healing around submerged and non-submerged dental implants in beagle dogs. J Periodontol 1999;70(3):248–254.

Glauser R, Ree A, Lundgren A, Gottow J, Hammerle CH, Scharer P. Immediate occlusal loading of Brånemark implants applied in various jawbone regions: a prospective, 1-year clinical study. Clin Implant Dent Relat Res 3(4):2001;204–213.

Glauser R, Ruhstaller P, Gottow J, Sennerby L, Portmann M, Hammerle CH. Immediate occlusal loading of Brånemark TiUnite implants placed predominantly in soft bone: 1-year results of a prospective clinical study. Clin Implant Dent Relat Res 2003;5(Suppl 1):47–56.

Grunder U. Stability of the mucosal topography around single-tooth implants and adjacent teeth: 1-year results. Int J Periodontics Restorative Dent 2000;20(1):11–17.

Hammerle CH, Chen ST, Wilson TG, Jr. Consensus statements and recommended clinical procedures regarding the placement of implants in extraction sockets. Int J Oral Maxillofac Implants 2004;19(Suppl):26–28.

Hardt CR, Grondahl K, Lekholm U, Wennstrom JL. Outcome of implant therapy in relation to experienced loss of periodontal bone support: a retrospective 5-year study. Clin Oral Implants Res 2002;13(5):488–494.

Hermann JS, Buser D, Schenk RK, Higginbottom FL, Cochran DL. Biologic width around titanium implants: a physiologically formed and stable dimension over time. Clin Oral Implants Res 2000;11(1):1–11.

Hermann JS, Buser D, Schenk RK, Schoolfield JD, Cochran DL. Biologic width around one- and two-piece titanium implants. Clin Oral Implants Res 2001;12(6):559–571.

Hermann JS, Schoolfield JD, Schenk RK, Buser D, Cochran DL. Influence of the size of the microgap on crestal bone changes around titanium implants: a histometric evaluation of unloaded non-submerged implants in the canine mandible. J Periodontol 2001;72(10):1372–1383.

Jokstad A, Braegger U, Brunski JB, Carr AB, Naert I, Wennerberg A. Quality of dental implants. Int Dent J 2003;53(6 Suppl 2): 409–443.

Kalk WW, Raghoebar GM, Jansma J, Boering G. Morbidity from iliac crest bone harvesting. J Oral Maxillofac Surg 1996; 54(12):1424–1429; discussion 1430.

King GN, Hermann JS, Schoolfield JD, Buser D, Cochran DL. Influence of the size of the microgap on crestal bone levels in non-submerged dental implants: a radiographic study in the canine mandible. J Periodontol 2002;73(10):1111–1117.

Klokkevold PR, Han TJ. How do smoking, diabetes, and periodontitis affect outcomes of implant treatment? Int J Oral Maxillofac Implants 2007;22(Suppl):173–202.

Lazzara R, Porter S, Testori T, Galante J, Zetterqvist L. A prospective multicenter study evaluating loading of osseotite implants two months after placement: one-year results. J Esthet Dent 1998;10(6):280–289.

Lazzara RJ, Testori T, Trisi P, Porter S, Weinstein RL. A human histologic analysis of osseotite and machined surfaces using implants with 2 opposing surfaces. Int J Periodontics Restorative Dent 1999;19(2):117–129.

Lincks J, Boyan BD, Blanchard CR, Lohmann CH, Liu Y, Cochran DL, et al. Response of MG63 osteoblast-like cells to titanium and titanium alloy is dependent on surface roughness and composition. Biomaterials 1998;19(23):2219–2232.

Martinez H, Davarpanah M, Missika P, Celletti R, Lazzara R. Optimal implant stabilization in low density bone. Clin Oral Implants Res 2001;12(5):423–432.

Misch CE. Progressive loading of bone with implant prostheses. J Dent Symp 1993;1:50–53.

Oh TJ, Yoon J, Misch CE, Wang HL. The causes of early implant bone loss: myth or science? J Periodontol 2002;73(3):322–333.

Piattelli A, Vrespa G, Petrone G, Iezzi G, Annibali S, Scarano A. Role of the microgap between implant and abutment: a retrospective histologic evaluation in monkeys. J Periodontol 2003;74(3):346–352.

Quirynen M, Van Assche N, Botticelli D, Berglundh T. How does the timing of implant placement to extraction affect outcome? Int J Oral Maxillofac Implants 2007;22(Suppl):203–223.

Raghavendra S, Wood MC, Taylor TD. Early wound healing around endosseous implants: a review of the literature. Int J Oral Maxillofac Implants 2005;20(3):425–431.

Roberts EW, Poon LC, Smith RK. Interface histology of rigid endosseous implants. J Oral Implantol 1986;12(3):406–416.

Rocci A, Martignoni M, Gottlow J. Immediate loading of Brånemark System TiUnite and machined-surface implants in the posterior mandible: a randomized open-ended clinical trial. Clin Implant Dent Relat Res 2003;5(Suppl 1):57–63.

Roser K, Johansson CB, Donath K, Albrektsson T. A new approach to demonstrate cellular activity in bone formation adjacent to implants. J Biomed Mater Res 2000;51(2):280–291.

Salinas TJ, Eckert SE. In patients requiring single-tooth replacement, what are the outcomes of implant- as compared to tooth-supported restorations? Int J Oral Maxillofac Implants 2007; 22(Suppl):71–95.

Schmitt A, Zarb GA. The longitudinal clinical effectiveness of osseointegrated dental implants for single-tooth replacement. Int J Prosthodont 1993;6(2):197–202.

Small PN, Tarnow DP. Gingival recession around implants: a 1-year longitudinal prospective study. Int J Oral Maxillofac Implants 2000;15(4):527–532.

Small PN, Tarnow DP, Cho SC. Gingival recession around wide-diameter versus standard-diameter implants: a 3- to 5-year longitudinal prospective study. Pract Proced Aesthet Dent 2001;13(2):143–146.

Smith DE, Zarb GA. Criteria for success of osseointegrated endosseous implants. J Prosthet Dent 1989;62(5):567–572.

Spear FM. Maintenance of the interdental papilla following anterior tooth removal. Pract Periodontics Aesthet Dent 1999;11(1): 21–28; quiz 30.

Spear FM, Mathews DM, Kokich VG. Interdisciplinary management of single-tooth implants. Semin Orthod 1997;3(1):45–72.

Tangerud T, Gronningsaeter AG, Taylor A. Fixed partial dentures supported by natural teeth and Brånemark system implants: a 3-year report. Int J Oral Maxillofac Implants 2002;17(2): 212–219.

Tarnow DP, Elian N, Fletcher P, Froum S, Magner A, Cho SC et al. Vertical distance from the crest of bone to the height of the interproximal papilla between adjacent implants. J Periodontol 2003;74(12):1785-1788.

Testori T, Meltzer A, Del Fabbro M, Zuffetti F, Troiano M, Francetti L, et al. Immediate occlusal loading of Osseotite implants in the lower edentulous jaw: a multicenter prospective study. Clin Oral Implants Res 2004;15(3):278–284.

Todescan FF, Pustiglioni FE, Imbronito AV, Albrektsson T, Gioso M. Influence of the microgap in the peri-implant hard and soft tissues: a histomorphometric study in dogs. Int J Oral Maxillofac Implants 2002;17(4):467–472.

Trisi P, Lazzara R, Rebaudi A, Rao W, Testori T, Porter SS. Bone–implant contact on machined and dual acid-etched surfaces after 2 months of healing in the human maxilla. J Periodontol 2003;74(7):945–956.

von Wowern N, Gotfredsen K. Implant-supported overdentures: a prevention of bone loss in edentulous mandibles? A 5-year follow-up study. Clin Oral Implants Res 2001;12(1):19–25.

Weber HP, Sukotjo C. Does the type of implant prosthesis affect outcomes in the partially edentulous patient? Int J Oral Maxillofac Implants 2007;22(Suppl):140–172.

Weng D, Jacobson Z, Tarnow D, Hurzeler MB, Faehn O, Sanavi F, et al. A prospective multicenter clinical trial of 3i machined-surface implants: results after 6 years of follow-up. Int J Oral Maxillofac Implants 2003;18(3):417–423.

Wennerberg A. Implant design and surface factors. Int J Prosthodont 2003;16(Suppl):45–47; discussion 47–51.

Wennerberg A, Albrektsson T. Suggested guidelines for the topographic evaluation of implant surfaces. Int J Oral Maxillofac Implants 2000;15(3):331–344.

277

Wennerberg A, Albrektsson T, Andersson B. Bone tissue response to commercially pure titanium implants blasted with fine and coarse particles of aluminum oxide. Int J Oral Maxillofac Implants 1996;11(1):38–45.

Wennerberg A, Albrektsson T, Andersson B. Design and surface characteristics of 13 commercially available oral implant systems. Int J Oral Maxillofac Implants 1993;8(6):622–633.

Wennerberg A, Hallgren C, Johansson C, Danelli S. A histomorphometric evaluation of screw-shaped implants each prepared with two surface roughnesses. Clin Oral Implants Res 1998;9(1):11–19.

Wiskott HW, Belser UC. Lack of integration of smooth titanium surfaces: a working hypothesis based on strains generated in the surrounding bone. Clin Oral Implants Res 1999;10(6):429–444.

Wright PS, Glantz PO, Randow K, Watson RM. The effects of fixed and removable implant-stabilised prostheses on posterior mandibular residual ridge resorption. Clin Oral Implants Res 2002;13(2):169–174.

Index